I0120292

The Sex Ed Playbook

Participatory Theatre for Health Education

by

Nik Zaleski, Jacob Watson,
Shannon Oliver-O'Neil, Alison Lehner,
Abby Zan, and Alyssa Vera Ramos

Copyright © 2022 Zaleski, Watson, Oliver-O'Neil, Lehner, Zan, and Ramos.
All rights reserved.
ISBN: 978-0-578-66490-3

"Play is grounded in the concept of possibility."
        - An Exploratory Model of Play, Csikszentmihalyi & Bennett

"In the measurement world, you set a goal and strive for it. In the universe of possibility, you set the context and let life unfold."
        - The Art of Possibility, Zander & Zander

CONTENTS

ABOUT THE AUTHORS

We are a group of artists, educators, and activists who worked together in Chicago from 2008 to 2014 developing theatre frameworks to improve sexual health practices. We founded and worked under the organization For Youth Inquiry (FYI): Performing Health Collective, with the mission to design participatory theatre experiences that activate the creative potential of health education. In 2014, FYI became a program of the Illinois Caucus for Adolescent Health (ICAH), an organization that educates and organizes for reproductive justice for youth in the state of Illinois. ICAH has a robust history of utilizing creative approaches to improve adolescent health, which are now infused with FYI's participatory theatrical practice. To learn more about ICAH's ongoing work in the reproductive justice movement, visit www.icah.org.

Throughout this book, we also draw from our individual experiences working with youth in theatre and health spaces as teaching artists, educators, activists, and advocates. We incorporate best practices from our collective work under FYI and years of bringing innovative cultural and theatre practice to the field of sexual health education. The authorship of this book intentionally mirrors our collaborative working style. And though you will hear from individual authors at points, the book is written with our collective voice at the helm.

Nik Zaleski is a facilitator, narrative artist, and intimate somatics coach who organizes her life around awe. She co-founded several social justice organizations and collectives that are still moving their impact through the world, including Ag47 Artist Mentorship Collective, Swarm Artist Residency, Shared Space, and her current organizational development company, Murmur. She has nearly two decades of experience working in social change movements, primarily for reproductive justice and sexual violence prevention. Artistically, she has directed dozens of participatory plays that move audiences to action and is currently a co-director of Sojourn Theatre. Nik also holds a BS in Gender Studies and Performance Studies from Northwestern University and an MA in Interdisciplinary Studies from DePaul University, where she combined Public Health and Theater Directing coursework in the MFA directing program.

Jacob Watson is a socially-engaged artist, researcher, and educator. He designs processes, plays, workshops, and programs that move people into deeper understanding of themselves and their communities. Jacob currently runs a freelance consulting practice focused on strategic planning and learning design. He is also the Director of Growth Stage Programming at UpStart, Research Associate and Learning Specialist at Convergence Design Lab, and an organizer for Swarm Artist Residency. Jacob has worked as a researcher at Project Zero and as a program manager for interdisciplinary learning initiatives at Columbia College Chicago's Center for Community Arts Partnerships. He has worked with a wide variety of cultural and educational institutions including Lyric Opera of Chicago, Redmoon, The Jewish Early Childhood Education Leadership Institute, Chicago Architecture Biennial, and Harvard's Bok Center for Teaching and Learning. Jacob received his EdM in Arts in Education from Harvard University and BA in Theatre from Northwestern University.

Shannon Oliver-O'Neil is a therapist, educator, and theatre maker. Her work focuses on the intersections of sexual and mental health. As a therapist, Shannon works with individuals and couples to improve sexual function and emotional health. As an educator, Shannon has created theatre-based curriculum for After School Matters, the Northwestern University Women's Center, Ag47, and the University of Michigan's Educational Theatre Company, which runs performance workshops on identity, community accountability, and bystander intervention for the Office of New Student and Parent Programs. She holds a BA in Theatre and Gender Studies from Northwestern University and an MSW from the University of Michigan.

Alison Lehner is a social worker, theatre artist, and educator. She hails from Chicago where she worked as a teaching artist and program director for multiple arts and social justice organizations. Most recently, Alison has worked as a clinical social worker with children and families in Chicago, the Bay Area, and Salt Lake City. She has a particular interest in attachment-based therapy, parent education, and personal wellness. She graduated from Northwestern University with a BA in Performance Studies and holds an MSW from Loyola University Chicago School of Social Work.

Abby Zan is an urban planner, researcher, and cultural worker committed to the collaborative, imaginative pursuit of more equitable, just, and sustainable places and systems. She is currently an Associate at WXY Studio, where she works with a wide range of clients, focusing on school planning, arts and cultural planning, and community engagement. Previously, Abby worked as the Connectivity Associate at Woolly Mammoth Theatre Company and as a Project Manager with Sheldon Scott Studios in Washington, DC. She has worked extensively as a teaching artist and facilitator. Abby holds an MS in Design and Urban Ecologies from Parsons School of Design and a BA in Performance Studies from Northwestern University.

Alyssa Vera Ramos is a cultural worker, facilitator, theatre artist, and organizer dedicated to dreaming — and living into — a liberated world. Alyssa has directed, devised, and co-written many plays and workshops for audiences of all ages. She serves as Artistic Director of For Youth Inquiry (FYI) Performance Company at Illinois Caucus for Adolescent Health (ICAH), where she directed and co-developed *Expectation* and supported new works, including *This Boat Called My Body* and *Sexuality Out Loud,* among others. Also of note is her work on the participatory *Epic Tales from the Land of Melanin*, selected for the Latinx Theatre Commons' International TYA Festival. As the former Director of Cultural Strategies at ICAH, Alyssa launched several legislatively successful cultural campaigns with youth, particularly for abortion access. She is a Curator of Swarm Artist Residency, focused on anti-racism and healing justice, and is the co-host of the podcast *Meeting Our Desires*. Alyssa holds a BS in Theatre from Northwestern University and is a graduate of the University of Michigan School of Social Work Sexual Health Certificate Program.

As we introduce ourselves, we want to take a moment to acknowledge the context within which we were able to write this book and develop the curriculum within it. As young artists eager to test our ideas, we were invited to teach in Chicago schools before any of us had significant credentials beyond our private undergraduate degrees. We were given the benefit of the doubt because many of us are white, all of us carry class privilege from our families, and because the Chicago Public School system's dearth of funding causes them to welcome contracted educators who offer enthusiastic and cheap labor. We were able to provide that cheap labor (working initially for free and later for low fees) because we had other means of income and support due to our privileges.

Many brilliant educators often hit obstacles that we did not. Many educators who are marginalized as a result of being young, broke, trans, Black, brown, or other disenfranchised identities are not granted access to teaching or arts-based positions that pay living wages, due in large part to systemic bias and oppression. Many folks do not have the luxury of being able to give away their skills or ideas for free, and indeed, should not be expected to. We continue to look to these innovators for insight on sexuality-related content delivery, and task our readers, especially those who hold privilege and/or power, to do the same. Similarly, the participatory nature of our curriculum is intended to make space to hear and honor those whose voices and talents are often marginalized by our society, and for facilitators with marginalized identities to be paid for their labor as they lead programs that utilize this work.

FOREWORD by Michael Rohd

What do you do when your students who are no longer your students invite you to write a foreword to a book they've written, and you say yes, and then, after multiple readings and deep reflection, you realize they wrote a better book than you did?

First, you talk about what you wrote: In 1996, I wrote a book called *Theatre for Community, Conflict and Dialogue: The Hope Is Vital Manual*. Heinemann Press published it in 1998. The book is based on a program I developed in Washington, DC, with teenagers and homeless men living with HIV/AIDS. I spent seven years partnering with communities to create versions of the program all over the United States, and my learnings became a manual for using theatre activities and processes to build space for challenging conversations in diverse settings with young people and adults. It still gets used a bunch.

Second, you talk about what you've done since then: In 1999, I founded an award-winning, ensemble-based theatre company called Sojourn Theatre. We make work around the United States. From 2007 to 2016, I was on faculty at Northwestern University where I met and taught each of the co-authors of this book (more on them soon). In 2011, I co-founded what is now a national organization called the Center for Performance and Civic Practice (CPCP) that supports the work of artists and communities working together to build arts-based, community-led transformation. And in summer 2016, I accepted the role of Institute Professor at Arizona State University's Herberger Institute of Design and Art, a new position that crosses disciplines and gives me the freedom to help invent and support campus, community, and national initiatives aimed at positive, equitable community health and development.

Then, third, you get back to the authors of this book:

Nik, Alison, Abby, Shannon, Alyssa and Jacob. Six of the smartest, most talented, passionate, and change-focused people I have had the honor to know, teach, and learn from. In the last eight years, they have started a theatre company dedicated to issues of youth and sexual health; they have managed the extraordinary feat of integrating that theatre company into a local organization that is dedicated to youth and health issues but was not previously an arts-centered space; they have built original performances, produced tours of these performances, and developed their own engaged pedagogy for change-aimed practice in diverse educational and youth settings; finally, they have turned their transformative youth practice into a deep commitment to trainings and tools for educators and health workers, so that their discoveries of how to radically, substantively improve the sexual health and classroom experiences of young people can impact as many youth as possible.

Fourth, you get to the important part: what they have accomplished with this book.

They have translated two key beliefs into a coherent, clear methodology with comprehensive, comprehensible activities, a legible, sensible framework, and advice throughout on implementation. Those two key beliefs? One: Shame has no place in the sexual education of young people (nor, for that matter, in education or engagement with youth in any context). And two: Theatre is a powerful tool for learning, for connection, for analysis, for joy, and for making vulnerable spaces and difficult dialogues safe and fruitful.

Fifth, you make it very clear why people should read this book: Because it is a remarkably and singularly accessible tool that you can use. There is complex thought in its construct, but an elegant and simple logic you can follow. There is depth in the journey it invites you to lead young people, but a lack of preciousness that will aid you in crafting the right experience for the youth who you know, care about, and engage. Whether you are a theatre artist, an educator, a youth worker, a health worker, leader of a peer education program, or youth advocate working with youth councils, this book will become a treasured resource.

What do you do when you realize your former students have written a better book than you did?

You proudly shout about it, hand it out wherever you go, and be thankful that from now on, you use it in your own work.

- Michael Rohd

Artist for Civic Imagination, Center for Performance and Civic Practice
Ensemble Member, Sojourn Theatre
Impact Advisor, One Nation/One Project
Institute Professor, Herberger Institute of Design and Art, Arizona State University

ACKNOWLEDGMENTS

Our work would not be possible without the mentorship and modeling of artists who have applied theatre practices in community spaces for decades. The list of people and places that championed this body of work range from youth groups to classroom teachers to devising theater artists and more. We are particularly indebted to the following:

Nicole Ripley, who co-created the first touring draft of *Project US,* providing the foundation and seeds for this project.

Michael Rohd, whose ongoing mentorship and early work in theatre-based HIV prevention continues to inspire this work.

Lys Sorresso, whose careful editorial eye helped to streamline the many voices and perspectives found in this text.

Jenni Kotting, who breathed life into these words with gorgeous design.

Vivian Piña, who gave the text a much-needed formatting makeover.

Past foundational collaborators, including Russell Love, Adam Welton, Adil Mansoor, Ariel Zetina, Aurelia Clunie, and Johanna Middleton.

The young women of Sisters Empowering Sisters at the Chicago Girls' Coalition, who co-developed many of the activities in this book.

Chicago Women's Health Center and Communities in Schools of Chicago for believing in this work in its early stages.

The Illinois Caucus for Adolescent Health (ICAH), which now houses new versions of participatory theatre methods that evolved from this book.

All Chicago-area youth who contributed their voices, stories, and imagination to our plays and activities.

A NOTE ON PRIMARY SOURCES

The tools in this book were inspired by a diverse set of applied theater practitioners who have worked in health and community contexts. We have done our best to trace the lineage of our approach (see *Participatory Theatre: a Blended Methodology*), while acknowledging the overlapping and uncertain origins of many of these ideas. Given the viral nature of theatre practices and their resistance to conventional forms of documentation, identifying the origin of many theater activities is like trying to uncover who invented the game of "tag." We know that Augusto Boal created Forum Theater. We know Dorothy Heathcote was the first to make circle drama forms accessible to drama educators. But spectrum activities, space walks, and character improvisations have been adapted by so many different theatre artists that it becomes difficult to locate their origins. Where possible, we have attempted to name and credit original sources.

Our work pulls most directly from theater practitioners Augusto Boal, Viola Spolin, Dorothy Heathcote, Michael Rohd, and Jan Selman. We are most influenced by the forms known commonly as "Creative Drama" and "Popular Theatre," whose historical origins we detail more closely in the methodology section. Throughout the Playbook, we have attempted to identify connections to these original sources. For each of the activities in Chapters 1 through 4, we offer "Connections" tags to help link our games and structures to these schools of thought and others.

We encourage you to check out our list of references in the back of the Playbook for connections to our primary inspirations and additional theatre artists. This effort seeks to connect our readers to a rich history of arts-based practices, as well as to lift up the work of our heroes. We have remixed and reworked their practices to best suit our audiences, and we hope you do the same in your own work.

WELCOME BACK: AN UPDATE FOR OUR TIMES

a note on touch, boundaries, bodies, adaptation, and our collective health:

In the time between the completion of this text and its publication, the world has been turned upside-down by the worst global pandemic of the last hundred years. For months, we were encouraged not to touch or be close to one another; not to gather in physical space; and to make countless other personal and public sacrifices to curb the spread of a dangerous virus.

At that time, in the spring of 2020, we were on the cusp of releasing this text into the world. Our author team made the difficult decision to delay publishing while we waited to see how long it would be before we could once again gather safely.

The activities in this book were designed to be led in-person: in classrooms and conferences, plazas and parks, and any other place people gather to learn about how to be good to each other and themselves. Now, as we near the end of 2021, we are finally starting to see the slow return of in-person programming. We believe that the time we've spent away from each other has only made the topics in this text even more relevant. For many people, COVID-19 provided a crash-course in boundaries and consent, a reminder that physical touch is not something to be considered lightly.

As we step tentatively into this new world, we must acknowledge the trauma many of us still carry from this pandemic time. Indeed, COVID-19 may be here to stay in one form or another, and no doubt many groups will be slow to re-integrate close contact, touch, and other forms of physical intimacy and activity into their work.

Let us be clear: All of the activities in this text can be facilitated without physical touch.

There are so many reasons to offer this adaptation. There have always been those for whom touch remains a complicated and contentious feature of a learning experience; and it's always a good idea to check in with groups about this before you begin. You might invite folks to meet one another, and themselves, with some simple breaths. You might ask that the group agree not to touch *at all* for the sake of simplicity, or you might invite a careful process of consensual touch that allows each person to set their own comfort level with physical contact. (If you pursue the latter, we encourage you to take your time to provide space for individual reflection before asking folks to state their boundaries out loud.)

We also recognize that we are living in a time of constant change. New developments in politics, climate, public health, and other spheres may call for additional adaptations of this work—whether in language, process, purpose, or context. As authors, we want to acknowledge the limited ability of our static text to anticipate such evolutions. Instead, we call on you, our contemporary reader, to embrace these ideas and activities as they best suit your place and time. After all, this is a book about creativity. And when the context shifts, we shift.

Welcome back, and thank you for joining us on this journey.

PREFACE

Why we wrote this book

More than ten years ago, while working with young people in arts- and community-based settings, we noticed something profound: Young people were eager to talk about sex and sexuality. And despite the amount of sexuality education these young people had received (or not received), confusion, shame, and stigma underscored their discussions and questions on the subject.

No matter the youth group's location, demographic, or stated objectives, the young people we encountered brought up issues related to sexuality:

- In a high school theatre ensemble, one boy continuously brought the topic of his virginity to the forefront of discussions about identity.
- As part of a leadership program for 14-to-20-year-old girls, simple group check-ins were riddled with insecurity around sexual experiences and budding relationships.
- When asked to write poems about their hopes for the future, high school students in one arts residency wrote about waiting to have sex until after college because they had learned that "you can't go to college with a baby."

None of the programs we facilitated back then intentionally sought out sexuality-related material. Yet the young people we worked with brought it to the table time and time again. We listened. Our curiosity as educators grew, and we began talking to one another, wondering why young people continued to bring these conversations up in arts-based settings.

The more we talked with the young people in these programs, the clearer the answer became: When it came to sex ed, the information they needed just wasn't there. Or when it was there, it didn't make room for the full nuance of who these young people were. It didn't prepare them for the range of creative approaches they might take in their path to navigating their own health and relationships.

So we looked for a new structure within which we could fully engage these questions about sexual health; something that actually incorporated youth voices and made space for the complexities of their experiences. Most importantly, we wanted something that wasn't just about delivering content; we wanted to help adults in schools become better allies and accomplices to youth.

With this goal in mind, we began to create performances and curricula, which we later called "participatory theatre" (a term whose history and usage is detailed more fully in the following introduction). In this process, we discovered that the very tools we had used in the past to devise performance content were great vehicles for education in and of themselves. We use the phrase "participatory theatre" in this text to refer to both the plays we created and toured and the accompanying collection of curricula and individual activities that we adapted for use in sexuality education contexts.

While our programs succeeded in opening the door for conversation, we began to notice that school staff were often too uncomfortable or ill-equipped to facilitate follow up discussions around issues of sexuality with their students. Although our programs were intended to complement existing sexual health curriculum, when asked about their sexuality education, we heard from our partners at schools that:

- Our plays provided the only sexual-health specific content students would encounter that year.
- Staff felt ill-equipped to answer basic sexual-health questions.
- When programs did exist, students invariably rated them as "awkward" and "scary."

Clearly, there wasn't just one problem here. Sex ed is complicated and hard to teach. Over the years, we worked with many great educators who found success in the classroom. But we also encountered educators who still struggled to communicate with their students in healthy and productive ways:

> *While touring our programs, we often worked alongside health teachers and other organizations tasked with providing sexuality education in schools. On one such occasion, a school nurse sat in on a performance to prepare for the continued discussion with students she would facilitate the next day. At the end of the play, she asked if she could contribute some "important information". She then directly addressed the girls (in a coed classroom) reminding them to be careful because "boys only want one thing, and will do ANYTHING to get it. And they don't have to deal with the consequences!" In that brief statement, the nurse managed to both cast all boys as sexual predators, and to cast all girls as potential victims. She reinforced the idea that boys don't face sex's less desirable consequences, and placed responsibility on girls for anticipating every potential move their*

partner makes rather than tuning into their own desire and communicating boundaries clearly. Not to mention the inherent heterosexism and presumption of the gender binary in the sentiment that all guys want girls and all girls want guys. Well-meaning as this nurse may have been, she hardly created a safe space to develop a sexual identity!
-Shannon Oliver-O'Neil

We discovered that the social fabric for talking and thinking about sexuality does not create an easy task for educators interested in promoting the health of young people. Adults like the nurse in Shannon's story don't shame young people for having sexual curiosities because they want them to feel bad about themselves, they do so because they are most familiar with fear-based methods that dominate the public health field. Indeed, many adults and educators have not yet imagined creative ways of exploring sexuality that dismantle fear and shame. Possibility for new education models often feels distant, and the charge to "save" young people from unintended pregnancy, STIs, and sexual violence feels urgent. This scarcity of creative mechanisms to talk and think about sexuality is a cultural problem.

We know that cultural problems demand cultural solutions. So we invented some.

Through years of sharing classrooms and prototyping activities together, we created a model for participatory theatre that addresses four anchor issues that regularly arise in sexuality education spaces. This model, called the 4 Ps, is designed as an antidote to some of the most common problems found in sexuality education:

- **PLEASURE:** Sex ed can be awkward, which prevents youth from enjoyable, open, and honest exploration of their experiences.
- **PERSPECTIVE:** Sex ed can be oversimplified to facts and data, making little room for complexity of experience and preventing youth from being able to critically examine different choices and scenarios.
- **PRACTICE:** Sex ed can be too afraid of failure, which prevents youth from trying out different ideas in order to learn what works in life.
- **POWER:** Sex ed can be too focused on dominant narratives, which prevents youth from accessing information that is relevant and inclusive of all perspectives and identities.

The model that emerged from these ideas compels and entices students into learning by affirming the value of **pleasure**, using **perspective** to encourage exploration of diverse perspectives, providing opportunities for **practice**, and encouraging a shared sense of **power** (more about this in the next section).

With this as our framework, we began to develop workshops for adult educators that used participatory theatre activities to help them imagine safe and accessible opportunities for their students to learn. Through the process of collaborating with educators, we built sustainable creative programming that affirms, normalizes, and supports youth sexual decision-making, and paves the road to healthier communities. Through the process of leading our adult-facing workshops with partner organizations and at conferences, we encountered more and more requests for resources. These requests motivated the creation of this book.

Although we created several touring participatory plays (scripted and performed by actor-facilitators), this book is not a guide for creating such a play. Rather this book focuses on the tools of participatory theatre themselves, and the ways they can be used to create curriculum and activate participation in your classroom, community center, youth group, etc.

Devising plays demands a different set of tools and processes, and we encourage you to check out the resources many other artists have already created on the subject. We mention some of them in our history of participatory theatre and others in our works cited.

Our aim is to provide both a theoretical model and practical guide. Youth workshops and work with educators are the core of this book. We begin this book by describing the need for innovative, arts-based strategies in sexuality education, and by positioning participatory theatre as a tool for cultivating empowering, engaging, youth-led learning environments. We then outline best practices in participatory theatre as well as over 40 different activities for use in a health context. Through sharing these applications and experiences, we hope to instill new vision, life, and creative energy into the field of youth sexuality education. We are eager to share tools with you, as you join us in reinventing the ways in which we teach young people about sexual health.

Who This Book is For
This book is for you—health workers, teaching artists, educators, youth and community advocates, or anyone seeking strategies to:

- Increase participant (youth or adult) participation in programs
- Create brave and innovative spaces for sexuality education

- Increase positive sexual health attitudes & behaviors

The activities provided in this book outline clear steps for facilitation and are designed to be flexible so that you can alter them to fit your individual style, needs, and approach.

As social practice artists, we have experimented with the activities in this book in wide-reaching contexts. From teaching artist residencies in schools and community spaces, to graduate study research projects, to therapeutic support groups, to performance workshops, we have seen them work in different spaces and with many audiences.

Many sexuality education curricula and trainings for healthcare professionals (such as evidence-based interventions and healthcare training modules) offer fully packaged sessions with activities that take the facilitator from start to finish. This book offers something different.

Our framework and activities can be used to create original curriculum or to supplement existing curriculum with participatory activities. This Playbook will show you a variety of ways to incorporate theatrical practice into your facilitation, whether or not you have experience.

We do incorporate basic sexual health content into activity descriptions. However, if you do not already have a grasp of this content, we suggest looking at some sexual health curriculum. Check out free *FLASH* sexuality curriculum or *Rights, Respect, Responsibility* from Advocates for Youth available online, or any of the following evidence-based curricula for accessible, well-packaged health information: *Our Whole Lives, Reducing the Risk,* and *Be Proud, Be Responsible*. We also love ICAH's comprehensive and inclusive curriculum, created in partnership with youth, S.L.A.Y.: Sexually Liberated and Affirmed Youth. Additional online resources include Sex, Etc. (www.sexetc.org) and Scarleteen (www.scarleteen.com), both targeted at youth audiences, and Planned Parenthood (www.plannedparenthood.com/learn).

How This Book is Organized
This book begins by describing the critical, pedagogical framework that underlines our work. We position participatory theatre as the key to unlocking the creative potential of sexuality education. In the text, we weave together anecdotal observations from personal experience in direct practice, alongside the history of theatre applied in a health and education context.

The subsequent chapters provide over 40 different participatory theatre activities for use in health education contexts. Aligned with the National

Sexuality Education Standards, our activities are organized around four goals: **Build Community, Share a Story, Move Your Body,** and **Act It Out.** The **Build Community** chapter offers game-based activities to cultivate a sense of community and trust within a group. The **Share a Story** chapter provides writing and storytelling activities to generate material or reflect on existing material. The **Move your Body** chapter presents physical activities to get participants out of their heads and moving into action. Finally, the **Act It Out** chapter uses role-play activities to help participants explore multiple perspectives and practice for real life scenarios.

INTRODUCTION

Why Participatory Theatre: A Case for Creative Sexuality Education

Creative sexuality education means thinking differently about how students construct understanding in the sexuality education classroom. In order to fully embrace the wide spectrum of possible perspectives around our own sexualities, we must inhabit a framework for learning that is built to sustain ambiguity, relativity, and flexibility.

What is participatory theatre?

an interactive, dialogical mode of performance, in which facilitators and participants co-construct and manipulate narratives through inquiry and play

---

In our work, we use the term **participatory theatre** to refer to our specific type of theatre practice. Similar to performances designed only for entertainment and spectacle purposes, participatory theatre uses performing and dramatic arts to engage the attention, interest, and curiosity of audience members[1]. But then, rather than seeking to explain, as in traditional educational and theatrical approaches, participatory theatre compares different life choices through role-play and character-led conversations, leading its audiences to engage in decision-making processes that position them as drivers of their own learning. We apply participatory theatre in a sexuality education context.

The reason our theatre is "participatory" is because we want the answers to come from the participants themselves. Too often, theatre used in educational settings becomes didactic, attempting to tell young people what they should believe or how they should behave. Not only is this ineffective and uninspiring to a young audience, it can actually serve to undermine, limit, and confuse their ability to make healthy decisions when circumstances differ from those presented in the performance (which, at some point, they inevitably will). Equally important, participatory theatre structures center and use the direct experiences and identities in the room.

When it comes to thinking and talking about sex, participatory theatre recognizes the multiplicity of values held by different people and communities. More traditional sexuality education practices might seek to apply a singular set of values among all students or apply a static definition for what is considered right and wrong. Rather than neatly solving the problem for them, this approach actually prevents students from understanding their own moral framework as it pertains to their sexuality.

A participatory approach diverges, not by denying that sex is linked to morality, but by encouraging participants to explore and form their own values, while thinking critically about where their deeply ingrained ideas about sex come from. These beliefs are influenced by culture, age, demographic, sexual orientation, geography, or religion. Participatory theatre in a sexuality education context moves beyond "right and wrong," and toward "right for you and right for me." Not only are there multiple "right" ways to think and act, but our sense of "rightness" can change, so "right for *you*" becomes "right for you *right now.*"

That said, there is no denying that some behaviors can be physically or emotionally harmful and should be avoided or reduced. As a general rule, we like to say that anything safe, consensual, and pleasurable is okay. Later in the introduction, we offer some general guidelines and best practices for holding these values while facilitating participatory theatre activities in a sexual health context.

Everyone brings different cultures, identities, and belief systems to the table. We all have different needs and values, as well as unique barriers to health, options, and decision-making. By intentionally infusing sexuality education with opportunities for authentic participation, these learning experiences can become truly "of" our participants, serving them in the way that is most useful. We've all seen theatre that tries too hard to tell its audience how to feel about a controversial topic (bullying, nutrition, and yes, sexuality), only to fall flat, with little to no impact.

Participatory Theatre: A Blended Methodology
Although the application of these kinds of theatre practices to sexuality education is relatively new, it is worth noting that the practices themselves have been around for some time. In fact, the phrase

"participatory theatre" has evolved as something of an umbrella term to refer to a wide variety of practices and concepts. In academic terms,

> *'Participatory Theatre' (PT) is used to cover practices referred to variously as Applied Theatre or Drama, Community Theatre, Workshop Theatre, Role Play etc. The practice ranges between work with a performance focus to process-based work aimed at personal group and/or social development. It takes place in a wide variety of employment, political, social and community settings and practitioners come from a variety of backgrounds. Practitioners may be professional theatre performers and directors, dedicated trained facilitators, or professionals from other backgrounds e.g. social work or education. Participatory theatre is internationally associated with radical and popular theatre forms such as Theatre in Education, Young People's Theatre, Forum Theatre (Theatre of the Oppressed), and Theatre for Development.[2]*

The field is vast. "Participatory Theatre" has come to refer to a diverse set of performance experiences. In order to distinguish this Playbook from the rest of the field, it is important to emphasize one truth: the brand of participatory theatre articulated here reflects processes, not plays. This Playbook outlines frameworks and exercises for learning experiences rather than scripts for staging.

Like many other participatory theatre practitioners, our work changes drastically depending on application context. The following pages will describe a methodology—a roadmap to healthy conversations about sexuality through participatory theatre techniques—rather than an end product. Thousands of different participatory theatre applications exist in the field, influenced by the participants and communities that each serve. We do not intend for the exercises outlined in this Playbook to speak monolithically to the whole field of participatory theatre, but rather to articulate our specific brand, heavily influenced by two distinct yet interrelated areas of practice: Creative Drama and Popular Theatre.

Creative Drama: Thinking From Within the Dilemma
While much contemporary practice in the field of participatory theatre tends toward political or civic outcomes, our particular brand of practice in this context leans educational. This should not be surprising, given our

collective theatre training in Evanston, Illinois, a city referred to in some circles as the "birthplace" of creative drama.

"Creative dramatics" (as it was originally called) refers to "an improvisational, non-exhibitional, process-oriented form of drama, where participants are guided by a leader to imagine, enact, and reflect on experiences real and imagined. Creative drama takes children's natural world, creative play, and develops it further, using theatre techniques, to create learning experiences which are for the participants."[3] We draw on this approach in our own work as we strive to empower participants to re-shape the narratives they have encountered around their own understanding of sexuality.

Winifred Ward: The "Mother" of Creative Drama

The advent of this field is largely credited to drama educator Winifred Ward, whose work at Northwestern University and in the local school district during the 1920s and '30s paved the way for the legitimacy of this practice as an approach to learning through story and imagination. Ward was inspired by progressive educator John Dewey's conceptualization of "learning by doing" and in 1930 had published her first book on this new educational methodology. Referred to similarly as "playmaking" or "dramatic play," Ward's approach sought to push back against the dullness of empty memorization and "ready-made plays" for children. The goal was not necessarily to create new plays with children; rather, Ward hoped that creative drama would afford the development of emotional and self-expressive qualities. "Drama is unique among the arts in its concrete use of people and social living as material," she writes. "Being many kinds of characters gives [the student] not only outlets for emotion but the chance to understand and discriminate among various ways of meeting situations."[4]

Viola Spolin: Getting Out of Our Heads

While Ward had worked initially as a public school teacher, other contributors to the field of creative drama — such as Viola Spolin — came from a background in community-based arts education. Originally hired as a drama supervisor with the Works Progress Administration (WPA) in Chicago in 1939, Spolin created the improvisational "theatre game," an influential play-based form that would eventually become the foundation for improv comedy troupes like the famed Second City.

During the 1940s, however (about 20 years before the birth of Second City), Spolin worked extensively with young people and found that theatre games were an effective way to cultivate spontaneity, authenticity, and creativity in rehearsal. These were active, on-your-feet games, which often involved components of character and story. Since then, theatre games have been applied in a variety of other settings to similar effect, including Spolin's 1986 text, *Theatre Games for the Classroom*. What is significant about Spolin's work is that it gave educators permission to play, to shift perspective, and to experience failure. These have become core tenets of theatre-based practice in the classroom and have had significant influence on our own framework, as we use games to break through some of the more challenging aspects of sexuality education.

Dorothy Heathcote: Negotiating Change

Like Ward, many early innovators of creative drama guided children in the acting out of familiar tales and stories. All that began to shift with the introduction of teachers like Dorothy Heathcote, whose "process drama" approach sought to use drama as a way to enhance the understanding of everyday, real-life scenarios. Fueled similarly by the promises of progressive education, as well as the political climate of the 1960s, Heathcote's approach in the United Kingdom was the first to employ what was known as "the mantle of the expert," a strategy that positioned learners as powerful and knowledgeable characters within the dramatic scenario.

For Heathcote, drama was a way of understanding how we navigate the world. In *Drama as a Process for Change*, she writes, "The most important manifestation about this thing called drama is that it must show change. It does not freeze a moment in time, it freezes a problem in time, and you examine the problem as the people go through a process of change." According to Heathcote, the dramatic arts offer an opportunity to enact behavioral change as a result of the imagined "interaction of people and forces," which "must be given a framework within which they negotiate their change, their interaction."[5] This framework refers to the structure of a dramatic scenario or activity, as it is used in a learning context.

Thus, the flexible nature of a dramatic scenario, which follows the artist's intuition rather than an external morality, frees individuals from fear of failure and enhances their sense of self-determination. It also allows us to actually embody our ideas, rather than to simply ponder them. As

Heathcote puts it, drama allows us to, "think from within the framework of choices, instead of talking coolly about the framework of choices."

In the last 40-plus years, the field of creative drama has exploded — both in the United States and internationally, leading to annual conferences, graduate programs, and professional development opportunities for classroom teachers. It is this legacy that we humbly build upon in our unique contributions to the field of sexuality education.

However, the story of our approach to participatory theatre would not be complete if we didn't mention another body of practice—a movement and methodology that radically shifted how theatre could be used toward the end of the 20th century.

Popular Theater: A Return to the People

Augusto Boal: From Spectator to Spect-actor

It would be impossible to describe the history of participatory theatre without referencing the work of Brazilian playwright and director, Augusto Boal, one of the founders of the Popular Theatre movement in the 1980s. Popular Theatre (literally, "of the people") emerged as a tool for the disenfranchised to look at societal and political issues of their own distinct communities within the safety of a fictitious world.[6] Augusto Boal developed the *Theatre of the Oppressed* pedagogy in which theatre is used as a language for oppressed and underrepresented groups and as a way to "rehearse for the revolution."

The Popular Theatre approach developed by Boal was, in part, a response to the type of theatre that told its audiences how to feel. Rather than a "spectator," Boal wanted an audience of "spect-actors"—audience members who would *act*, who would take part in the formation of the story and influence its outcome. Boal's *Theatre of the Oppressed* casts the spectator as no longer delegating power to the characters to act in their place. They are free to act and think for themselves, because theatre is action.

During his career, Boal invented several theatre forms that popular theatre artists still utilize today.[7]

Forum Theatre is Boal's most popularized form, which offers a scene where a spect-actor can freeze to replace the protagonist and interrupt the oppression.

Invisible Theatre performs a scene in an environment other than a theater (like a restaurant, sidewalk, train, etc.) for audiences who are there by chance. The scenes are meant to be "invisible" as theatre, meaning that audiences should read them as reality with the aim of eliciting some action from them.

Image Theatre is a performance technique in which one person, acting as a sculptor, molds other performers acting as statues, using only touch.

Legislative Theatre, iterated primarily in Boal's last years of life, allows voters to voice their opinions on proposed laws to be passed.

Newspaper Theatre consists of several simple techniques for transforming daily news items, or any other non-dramatic material, into theatrical performances.

Rainbow of Desire builds on image theatre techniques and focuses on internalized experiences of oppression.

Augusto Boal's work has made significant contributions to participatory theatre companies and practices across the globe. While his frameworks and applications vary from context to context, *Theatre of the Oppressed* has impacted every theatre artist attempting to move their audiences beyond passivity and toward action.

(A note: Readers who are familiar with Boal's work will notice that we offer an adapted application of these techniques. In traditional Theater of the Oppressed and Forum theater exercises, for example, the "oppressor" role is not swapped out, nor is their transformation the subject of interest. Actors, instead, swap in and out for the "oppressed" characters, trying on strategies to dismantle systemic injustices. Our adaptations blend aspects of creative drama practice, making space for actors to swap in and rehearse changes for both roles. You'll see this adaptation in 4-3: Transforming Oppressive Messages, and throughout Chapter 4.)

Paulo Freire: Education As the Practice of Freedom

Boal's work and life was inspired by radical educator Paulo Freire, who created a model of learning that posited that audiences could use education to take power into their own hands. Freire first called for a liberatory model of education in the early 1970s, insisting that students be seen as active participants in the construction of knowledge and not empty vessels to be filled with ideas. Freire posed that learning stems from the place of individual knowledge and wisdom and that learners should be active participants in sharing their expertise. "The teacher," he said, "cannot think for her students, nor can she impose her thought on them. Authentic thinking . . . does not take place in ivory tower isolation, but only in communication."[8] Freire's work demanding that learners be active participants in knowledge creation and dissemination is an essential pedagogical foundation for participatory theatre.

Bertolt Brecht: Resisting Catharsis

Boal was also deeply inspired by the work of German theatrician Bertolt Brecht, who popularized the 'alienation effect' in playmaking. For Brecht, the theater was a place where audiences should go to think (and hence, prepare for action), rather than experience the high levels of emotional catharsis that so much of the theatre of his time put attention toward. For this reason, his *Verfremdungseffekt*, or alienation effect, was meant to make the familiar strange by drawing the audience's attention to contradictions in society.[9] Brecht rallied against the idea that the theatre was a place where audiences should go to passively receive creative material that helped them forget the world they lived in. He wanted a thinking, *active* audience, a perspective that anchored him as one of the primary founders of participatory theatre.

Interactive Theatre

While often used interchangeably with "participatory theatre," interactive theatre refers to any type of performance in which the audience is invited to take part in the action onstage. Unlike Popular Theatre, interactive theatre may or may not have revolutionary, or even politically-motivated, aims. Some forms of interactive theatre, such as **Playback theatre** (in which professional actors improvise a story based on the real lives of audience members), have a history of use in more therapeutic contexts.[10]

Sometimes the concept of an "audience" is removed entirely. **Immersive theatre**—in which the audience is literally enmeshed in the performance space alongside the actors—has a long history in Europe and has grown steadily in the United States since the early 2000s.

While practices like these "activate" the audience in ways that are apparently and structurally similar to the "spect-actor" of Popular Theatre, it is important to note that these experiences are not necessarily designed to meet the same ends. Some scholars have begun to critique certain forms of interactive theatre for offering a pretense of audience "freedom" veiled by a highly-restrictive menu of interactive options.[11] In other words, the autonomy of the participant is not always a primary goal.

Still, some forms of interactive theatre are explicitly educational, such as **theatre-in-education**, which is used to describe experiences in which professional actors tour schools with pre-made plays that include moments of designed interaction built into the experience. Again, while we use the term "participatory theatre" to refer primarily to a *process* of co-constructing ideas through interaction, one could certainly use the activities in this book—as we have in other contexts—to build out scripted performances that engage learners in a similar way.

Drama? Theatre? Whose term is it anyway?
At this point, we have named a variety of practices that have shaped the way we think about the use of performance as a methodology within the context of sexuality education. It is worth acknowledging here that each of the people who have influenced us describes their work in a slightly different way.

While many educators use the word "drama" to distinguish their process-based approach from formally producing plays, we have chosen the term "participatory theatre" to reflect both the artfulness of our practice and the significant influence of popular theatre, which we blend with traditional educational methodologies like creative drama.

In truth, the two words are relatively interchangeable. "Drama" tends to be used more in educational spaces, whereas professional companies and, increasingly, action researchers, are likely to refer to their practice as "theatre" or "applied theatre." There are also regional differences.

At the end of the day, our goal is simply to chart the course of our own methodological development and to pay tribute to the leaders who inspired us to use the tools of theatre in service of personal learning and growth. We hope that you will follow our example in borrowing, blending, and building upon these ideas, in whatever way best suits your own unique context.

Authentic Participation: Moving Beyond Engagement

One important quality that connects each of these leaders is their belief in people's ability to drive their own learning experience. Whether the learners were young children in a grade-school classroom or farmworkers in Brazil, valuing each person's ideas and autonomy was a core feature of each approach.

When we talk about participation in learning, we often hear the phrase "student engagement." Educational performances are frequently hailed for their ability to "engage" students in learning. But we must be wary of setting engagement as our end goal. While it is true that engagement can be productive, it doesn't always go far enough. *Engagement* means that participants are doing what you've asked, and perhaps they are even enjoying themselves or making meaningful contributions. (Certainly this is a step above *compliance*, the simple act of doing a task at a base level in order to avoid punishment or shame.)

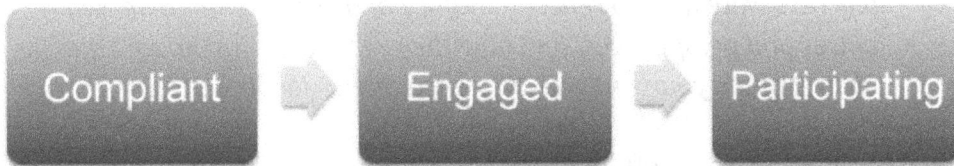

Compliant		Engaged		Participating

But if we allow ourselves to stop with engagement, we will never experience the genuine wisdom and guidance that youth voices can offer. *Participation* means players are a part of a whole—and that the whole cannot exist without the meaningful action of all involved. When we refer to our technique as *participatory*, we are talking about a mutually-supported, shared effort to create, learn, and explore. In a truly effective participatory invitation, facilitator and participant are making decisions and participating together, side-by-side. This is especially important when working with youth or other disenfranchised groups. Too often, learning experiences are designed without the input of those they are meant to serve. By sharing power, we recognize the expertise that these populations bring, and respect their role as co-creators in the process.

When we explore sexuality through this kind of framework, we come to understand the relativity of our own sense of right and wrong. When we see our own biases, assumptions, and misconceptions more clearly, we are better prepared to move through the awkwardness and confusion of not knowing. Participatory theatre structures a framework of *"right for you right now,"* and sets the stage for a genuine moment of understanding across perspectives.

> *I remember facilitating a workshop at one of our partner schools for a group of teachers who wanted to learn how to better support these types of conversations with young people. We were doing an improvisation around questions their students had asked, and I was in the role of a student asking about whether it was the "right time" to have sex. My scene partner, a teacher at the school, offered the best response she could come up with: "Wait until you're older. You don't need to be thinking about that right now. You should focus on your schoolwork." While entirely well-meaning, this teacher's response had just undermined my character's ability to make an informed, personal decision about his sexual behavior. We paused the activity to debrief this scenario, and discuss the impact of that response. In this way, the teachers were able to reflect mindfully and critically on their own biases and perspectives, and how their responses can impact the agency of the young people they encounter. - Jacob Watson*

Theatre allows us to carefully examine a moment in time, and reflect critically upon our choices. Here, we draw primarily on the work of Heathcote and Boal, both of whom saw theatre as a site of inquiry as well as action. Healthcare providers, educators, and all adults who care about young people can look to participatory theatre to create an environment that makes room for multiple narratives and possibilities within a challenging and contentious topic.

Game + Story = Participatory Theatre

Our particular brand of participatory theatre is a combination of **game** and **story.**

Through the improvisational blend of these two forms, our process of participatory theatre makes space for all possible scenarios and points of view. When we engage in this kind of improvisational framework through theatre, we restore agency and decision-making power around health content to young participants. Rather than imposing an external morality of our own, we create a space in which young people can make the best choices for themselves, while equipped with factual information, and the framework of "safe, consensual, and pleasurable."

Storytelling strategies carry abundant benefits for health education. At its core, story provides multiple opportunities for empathy and critical reflection. When facilitators use storytelling strategies in sexuality education, they help young people understand non-dominant and diverse experiences that may connect to their own, and in these moments of connection, shame is reduced. Unique from other educational strategies, story supports youth in their identity formation by casting them as protagonists in their own lives. Telling our stories—real or imagined—can break down barriers and challenge the dominant narratives that surround us.

The process of enacting stories as an educational tool is timeless. Young people and adults have been telling, recording, reading, and performing stories in learning spaces for centuries. Stories are essential to how we make sense of the world around us, and in this aspect of our work we continue to be inspired by Ward and her contemporaries in the field of creative drama. We draw on this legacy in our own work, as we strive to empower participants to re-shape the narratives they have encountered around their own understanding of sexuality.

> *I remember facilitating an activity in a classroom in which the youth were not particularly well supported by the adults in their lives around their sexuality. The task at hand was to create improvised scenes inspired by the group's real, difficult-to-answer questions. Two student volunteers confidently and thoughtfully suggested a scenario: a student approaches a teacher at a quiet moment during lunch and asks about local sexual health resources. I remember the student playing the teacher in the scene as attentive and generous, fully present with the student's experience and curiosity. In that moment, the students were doing more than playing with perspective and fulfilling the demands of the exercise. They were proposing a new narrative—for their classroom and for their world. - Abby Zan*

Like stories, **games** offer several distinct functions that can bolster the agency and improve the health of young people. First, games help groups connect to each other, bond, and form a cohesive community. Building community in this way is critical in the process of moving through awkwardness and apprehension. Games help us cultivate joy, which in turn increases our willingness to accept future invitations to participate.

Games help youth:
- Define social norms and identity
- Negotiate the risks of the adult world without fear of failure
- Develop group identity and cohesion
- Dream and plan utopian revisions of the world
- Practice for real life
- Get in "flow" (more on this concept below)
- Experiment and transgress

> *Throughout my work in adolescent sexuality education, I watch youth openly and freely explore complex emotions and ideas with near-strangers when asked to play games. In the first fifteen minutes of an orientation for a youth leadership program I ran, youth who had never met before shared deeply personal stories about their aspirations and fears with each other because they were asked to do so in the context of freeze tag. The youth reflected to me months later that they felt closer to each other in that fifteen minute game of tag than they felt to their peers after a year of sharing classroom space together. - Nik Zaleski*

Being inside the chaos and order of a game like freeze tag not only helps players connect with one another in meaningful ways, but also gets them in "flow." True for both youth and adults, this concept suggests that one can be so absorbed by creative activity that ego and self-consciousness fall away.[12]

Play also frees young people from fear of failure and helps them negotiate the risks of the adult world with perspective as a buffer. Just as games teach young people about rules and processes, they also help youth understand when and how to break those rules by encouraging experimentation and transgression.[13] Societal rules and expectations aren't always set up for young people to succeed, especially those who hold socially stigmatized identities like houseless, transgender, and/or youth of color. These young people especially need to experiment with safe rule-breaking, which can move them out of dominant societal expectations that don't meet their needs.

Of course, there are many different types of "games," and our brand of game is particularly active, on-your-feet, and often involving components of character and story. This idea of a "theatre game" originated from a series of acting exercises developed by Spolin and expanded upon by many others along the way. These games have become core tenets of theatre-based practice in the classroom and have had significant influence on our own framework, which we refer to as the "4 Ps of Participatory Theatre."

The "4 Ps" of Participatory Theatre

Our style of participatory theatre offers a model that compels and entices students into learning by providing affirmation of **pleasure**, an exploration of a diversity of **perspective** (including one's own), opportunities for **practice**, and a shared sense of **power**. In combination, these elements uniquely activate the creative potential of sexuality education spaces.

First, participatory theatre affirms the value of **pleasure** in the learning environment. While pleasure may seem like a risqué word to use when talking about a classroom, it isn't. The truth is that understanding the importance of pleasure is a critical part of recognizing the role of sex, sexuality, and sensuality in our lives. We want students to recognize that just as learning can be silly, playful, and spontaneous, so too can they approach their sexuality with freedom and curiosity. In our model, we seek to create pleasurable learning experiences through the use of games, stories, and humor. This invigorates the classroom experience, helping youth laugh, enjoy, and follow their intuition. It can also help content feel more accessible, less overwhelming, and improve the ability of youth to stay in difficult conversations for longer periods of time. Also, in a pleasure-centered theatre practice, no ideas fail, and a sense of creative freedom follows, which enables students to engage more fully in classroom spaces. Because of this freedom, students take more risks and can make more self-driven discoveries.

Participatory theatre also provides opportunities to explore the **perspectives** of myriad people and sources. In educational spaces, the inclusion of others' perspectives functions as a tool for learning and positive decision-making, as participants help make choices about characters in their stories; engaging with those characters as they make decisions provides models for youth to live by or depart from.[14] Participatory theatre also explores diverse perspectives by teaching empathy, as participants must evaluate and affirm a multiplicity of stories. Since youth receive countless messages about how to behave sexually, about who to want and what to question, exploring non-dominant perspectives is particularly critical in developing healthy sexuality.

Additionally, participatory theatre provides the opportunity to **practice** for real-life decision-making: like how to ask for consent, or respond to an oppressive message from a parent. If acting is doing, then enacting positive communication styles and sexuality-related behaviors also prepares youth to "do" those actions in real life. Practice presents students with the opportunity to try on authentic, real-life examples for problem solving. In this way, participatory theatre provides safe opportunities to practice decision-making strategies and enact potential outcomes without fear of failure. This enables participants to prepare for similar situations in their daily lives.

Finally, participatory theatre disrupts **power** dynamics in learning by casting educators and students as co-participants. Democratic education manifests when facilitators and teachers model risk-taking for their students, a common occurrence when using theatre games, for example. Educators and learners meet each other on the same plane and share power that is ordinarily reserved for the teacher alone.[15] It is on this plane that discoveries happen, through educator and learner collaboration, where both depend on each other to succeed. Participatory theatre cannot function without youth voice and participation. Because youth direct the objectives of participatory plays and games, they experience braver and bolder engagement. The disruption of power dynamics breaks traditional classroom expectations by denouncing expertise and casting learners as educators.[16] The use of democratic education leads to less manipulative dialogue, and, instead, to authentic learning that gives power to and prioritizes the motivations and needs of each learner.[17]

Every activity in this Playbook uses the "4 Ps" of participation: Pleasure, Perspective, Practice, and Power. Elements of **pleasure** offer vitality and enjoyment to educational spaces, and invigorate curriculum. Exploration of diverse **perspective** presents low-risk ways for participants to share their own experiences through the safety of character. Opportunities to **practice** help participants put their education and knowledge to work in a safe space without fear of failure, preparing for future situations and conversations. And equally shared **power** in these activity structures facilitates a meaningful, intentional, and equitable exchange of ideas between educators and learners. As a facilitator, keep the 4 Ps in mind to assist you in creating a bold and thriving learning environment for your participants.

How to Use These Activities

As you approach the following chapters, we invite you to take a moment to think about your practice as it currently exists:

1. What already works well?
2. Where do you struggle to make connections or convey information?
3. Are there topics that you (or your participants) avoid?
4. What feels most challenging?
5. Where do you find the most joy?
6. If you are new to this work, what do you hope to discover through this process?

Consider the answers to these questions as a touchstone for how this book can serve your unique needs. We encourage you to use this Playbook in whatever manner is most helpful to you. Each activity comes with complete step-by-step instructions to lead you through even the most difficult content. Additionally, you'll find tips and tricks for successful facilitation at the end of this chapter, which you can apply to any scenario. Words in bold appear in our glossary.

The activities that follow are coded and organized in three ways: 1) **activity type**, 2) **level of exposure**, and 3) **content tag**. Use these markers to help you decide which activities are going to best fit your needs and interests.

Activity Type: What the activities DO.
The activities that follow are broken down into four chapters by **activity type**:

1. **Build Community**: Use these game-based activities to cultivate a sense of community and trust within your group.
2. **Share a Story**: Use these writing and storytelling activities to find common experience or reflect on existing ideas.
3. **Move Your Body**: Use these physical activities to get participants out of their heads and moving into action.
4. **Act It Out**: Use these role-play activities to help participants explore multiple perspectives and practice for real-life scenarios.

The activities in each chapter appeal to different learning styles. We invite you to weave activities from different chapters into your curriculum to cultivate designed, meaningful, and varied invitations to participate. However, this is not a necessity. There may be times when you want to lead a 90-minute session using only writing activities, for example, if this is appropriate for your group of participants and objectives. Follow your own intuition here, and choose the activities that best suit your purpose.

Levels of Exposure: How INTENSE the experience is.
A fundamental element to consider when choosing activities is the participants' **level of exposure,** or the amount of attention received from other learners during play. We encourage a strong consideration of level of exposure in order to intentionally arrange activities so that players move from lower to higher level forms of engagement carefully and successfully. We choose to structure activities in this way for the same reason swimming lessons never begin in the deep end, but start in shallow water. Therefore, the activities in each **activity type** are further broken down into three sections: low, medium, and high exposure. This is indicated by the three gray bars:

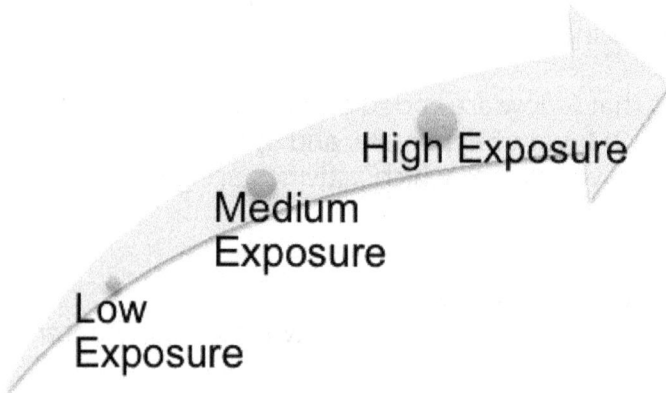

High Exposure

Medium Exposure

Low Exposure

The primary differences between low, medium, and high exposure activities can be understood based on qualities of **visibility**, **choice**, and **stakes**.

EXPOSURE	Low	Medium	High
Visibility	Big group, everyone plays together	Some play while others watch, equal opportunity to opt in or out	Small number of people (or 1 person) plays, watched by the rest of the group
Choice	Lots of choice, different ways to engage	2-3 different ways to engage, curated by facilitator	No choice, only 1 way to play or 1 thing to do/read/say
Stakes	Impersonal or low-stakes content: Someone else's story, or no story	Combination of personal and impersonal, or ability to associate one's own story with someone else's	Personal: Exposing a personal opinion, experience, or value in front of the group
Example: "Word Association"	*"On the count of three, everyone simultaneously call out one word you associate with love, dating, or sex."*	*"Everyone, go around the circle and individually say one word you associate with sex, or 'pass' if you can't think of one."*	*"One at a time, say one word you associate with sex and share a story about why that word came to mind."*

Content Tags & Standards Alignment: What the activities are ABOUT.
Each activity also includes a **content tag**, which will help you to plug activities into existing sexuality curriculum, or build original curriculum from the ground up based on a specific topic. Each activity is coded for at least one content tag that best describes the sexuality and/or health topic addressed.

These content tags align with the National Sexuality Education Standards (NSES) created by the Future of Sex Education (FoSE).[18] While we did not align individual activities with a specific NSES, the activities are intentionally crafted to address multiple content areas and topics. Just as we encourage flexibility in the facilitation of these methods, we invite multiple applications for the activities. For instance, though our work roots these games in the world of adolescent health, you can use them as containers for myriad social-emotional topics. See below for more on how our six content tags map to various NSES standards:

Start The Convo (on starting health-centered dialogue)

Start The Convo activities open the door to safe, accessible conversations about sexuality. They cultivate honest, shame-free dialogue about difficult or taboo topics. Use these activities in tackling any health topic for the first time, as they are intended to catalyze initial conversations rather than continue existing narratives. Start The Convo games spark engagement and cultivate inquiry around a topic.

These activities map to many of the NSES Interpersonal Communication (IC) standards, which help students develop interpersonal communication skills to enhance health and/or avoid health risks.

Health-411 (on health-related information)

Health-411 activities explore an array of sexuality topics that parallel National Sexuality Standards including, but not limited to: Anatomy, puberty and development, sexually transmitted infections (STIs) including HIV, and methods of contraception. Use these activities to examine health information and facilitate knowledge acquisition on specific health topics.

These activities map to many of the NSES Accessing Information (AI) standards, which help students access valid information, products, and services that enhance health, as well as the Core Concepts (CC) standards, which lead students to comprehend concepts related to health promotion and disease prevention.

<u>A word about teaching STI content:</u> It is important to speak about STIs in particular in a factual, objective way, steering clear of opinions, judgments, and words like "clean" (which implies that folks with STIs are "dirty"). This is one way you can strive to include everyone in conversations about safer sex, without potentially isolating or causing unintended harm to students who have experienced STIs and/or students born HIV-positive.

Does That Count? (on healthy relationships, warning signs and sexual violence)

Use these activities to help participants question what "counts" as sexual violence when they encounter problematic messages and behaviors in their world. *Does That Count?* activities analyze examples and root causes

THE SEX ED PLAYBOOK

of sexual violence. These activities help participants identify instances of sexual violence while developing action plans to interrupt and respond. In recognizing sexual violence in their lives and communities, participants will also understand how to create healthier interpersonal and institutional relationships.

These activities map to many of the NSES Interpersonal Communication (IC) standards as well as the Decision-Making (DM) standards, which help students develop the ability to use decision-making skills to enhance health.

Me/We (on identity, boundaries and goal-setting)

Me/We activities investigate individual identity in a social context, including but not limited to: Sexual orientation, gender identity and expression, personal boundary setting, and one's internal sense of sexuality based on race, class, gender, age, ability, etc. These activities create a safe space for participants to analyze social determinants of their own identity, set goals, and position themselves as the protagonists in their own lives.

These activities map to many of the NSES Goal Setting (GS) standards, which help students set goals to enhance health, as well as the Self-Management (SM) standards, which help students practice health-enhancing behaviors, and avoid or reduce health risks.

Bigger Than Us (on examining systems and influences)

Use these activities to lead participants in deeper understanding of systemic issues that are *Bigger Than Us*. Participants will examine institutional change processes by thinking beyond the interpersonal level. They will consider the effects of various influences in their lives, and infer ways to embrace or reject the power of those influences.

These activities map to many of the NSES Analyzing Influences (INF) standards, which help students analyze the influence of family, peers, culture, media, technology, and other factors in health behaviors.

Take Action (on advocacy and activism)

Take Action activities help participants achieve what Augusto Boal called "rehearsal for revolution." They provide safe space to practice interrupting oppressive practices and policies. Use these activities to help participants *Take Action* and respond to a spectrum of injustices from microaggressions to historical, systemic oppression.

These activities map to many of the NSES Advocacy (ADV) standards, which help students advocate for personal, family, and community health.

<u>A note on age-appropriateness:</u> The activities in this book were designed primarily for high school and college-age participants, with some activities for a middle-school age-range. The National Sexuality Education Standards outline core topics by age group, ranging from grades K-12. If you are uncertain about whether an activity is appropriate for your age demographic, consult the NSES, available free online at www.futureofsexed.org.

Activity Depth Tags: *How long and complex the activities are.*

The activities are also tagged according to their length and complexity. Please note that our time estimates will vary according to the size of your group. Look for the icons below to decide how much time to set aside for an activity.

Quick Dip
These activities are simple to set up, and do not take much time to play. They make great warm-ups, transitions, or closing moments. **Allot 5 to 10 minutes**.

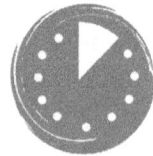

Short Swim
These activities are a bit more involved than the Quick Dips, but also do not require much set-up. Plan for more set-up and processing time. **Allot 10 to 15 minutes**.

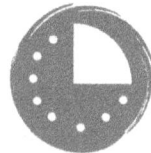

Jump In
These activities generally require a fair amount of set-up. They are either scaffolded to involve a number of different steps, or present a complex challenge or opportunity that calls for more time and deeper attention. **Allot 15 to 30 minutes**.

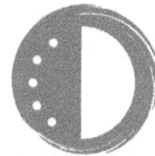

Deep Dive
These activities are the most complex and time-consuming in our collection. It is possible to build an entire class session around one of these activities. **Allot 30 minutes to an hour**.

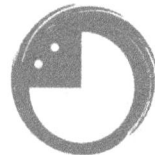

How to Design Your Curriculum

Keeping the *Activity Type, Level of Exposure,* and *Content Tag* in mind, we suggest structuring the activities of this Playbook for your facilitation in one of the following ways:

Build original curriculum
When using the Playbook to design curriculum from the ground up:

- Select activities with content tags that address your topic of choice.
- Ensure inclusion of activities from various chapters/activity types.
- Arrange activities from low to high exposure.

Appendix B offers a number of suggested 'activity playlists' or curated curriculum sessions. Refer to this section for ideas on how to structure your original curriculum, or start by trying out one of our 'playlists' with your students.

Supplement existing curriculum
When using the Playbook to supplement existing curriculum with participatory activities, consider the following questions:

- What level of exposure does my existing curriculum use?
  - *If High Exposure:* What low-exposure activities in the Playbook could lead learners to feel more comfortable participating in my existing curriculum?
  - *If Low Exposure:* What high-exposure activities could be applied to push learners to engage more fully, thoughtfully, and in more challenging ways?
- *What learning styles does my existing curriculum address?* Which gaps do I need to fill in? Use <u>activity type</u> (building community, writing, movement, acting) to address these other styles of learning.
- *What subject areas are already covered?* What is missing? Use <u>content tags</u> to help fill in gaps in your curriculum and cover all necessary or desired topics.
- Choose supplementary activities from there.

This Playbook offers activities in this format to intentionally ignite you as a participant and co-designer of curricula. The activities that follow are strongest when woven together to address various learning styles, multiple levels of exposure, and targeted content. Each activity can be arranged and adjusted for different ages or other group demographics.

We trust that you know your community of learners and invite you to organize activities in the way that suits them best.

Facilitation in a Participatory Theatre Context

The activities of this Playbook can be led in a variety of ways, and we expect you will bring your own facilitation style and approach to the work. For a few of the more complex activities (*1-4, 2-13, and 3-6*) we have provided *sample facilitation scripts* to help you get started.

Below are some additional guidelines that have helped us find success in leading participatory theatre activities in a sexuality education context:

1. **Recognize and acknowledge the identities that you as a facilitator bring to the space.**

Sharing power with participants is an ongoing practice, and something that requires consistent attention. Facilitators *do* bring power dynamics into the room: You may be choosing to be there, while others may be required to; you may be getting paid, while participants may not be. Regardless, you are coming into the space with certain knowledge and experiences that the participants you engage may not have (although they are experts in their own experiences). It's important to acknowledge these identities as a first step toward building trust and rapport around what can be sensitive subject matter.

To that end, it is also important to be conscious of if and how your identities—including identities others may perceive you to have (i.e., based on your skin color or your status as an authority figure) differ from the population you are serving. Sometimes, it may be important to explicitly state these differences. Sometimes, not. We encourage you to consider your class, gender, race, sexual identity, language, citizenship status, etc. and to be open to using these differences to talk about power systems, intersectionality, diversity, and communication with your participants when appropriate.

2. **Set up clear rules and expectations**

Even when we are playing, we need structure. Let your participants know how an activity is going to unfold, what they will or won't be asked to do, and what kinds of behaviors and ideas are or aren't allowed. Make room for the positive, too. We see young people react with surprise when we tell them they are allowed to say "any word" (even a "dirty" word) during our improvisational games. So often young people are told what not to do, that sometimes telling them they *can* do or say something is a revelation.

3. Create opportunity for opt-out

Not every one of your participants is going to be comfortable with every activity you introduce. It is likely that there will be moments when somebody needs to opt-out of an activity for some reason; they may become overwhelmed, exhausted, embarrassed, or any number of reactions. This is okay. These activities can be difficult at times. Encourage your participants to be in charge of their own bodies, and create space for them to disengage when necessary. Remind your group that there are many different ways to participate and that, as long as they are not distracting others from the experience, they have a right to engage in whatever way feels safe for them.

It can be helpful to offer guidelines to participants who may need to opt-out of an activity. Introduce these in advance, so that they are easy to apply whenever discomfort may arise:

1) Keep breathing
2) Turn discomfort into inquiry
3) Keep your attention focused in the room[19]

4. Don't tell them what they are going to learn

One of the easiest ways to sabotage an activity is to begin by explaining what you hope participants will know or understand as a result of their engagement. Do not do this. Instead, say just enough so that participants understand how to engage and what the goals are. Let them discover the greater meaning or significance through doing. Then, guide a reflection following the activity where the participants can share their discoveries and responses. Learning is not a secret, but even you may be surprised by the outcome of each activity.

5. Let the group guide the conversation

Sometimes you may walk into a room intending to shape the conversation in a certain way, or you may choose a certain activity hoping that a particular topic or dialogue will spark. Be sensitive to the group's interests, and allow the conversation to go where it wants to. This approach almost always results in a richer, more dynamic, and more useful dialogue than one that was premeditated by the facilitator.

Additionally, every game will affect each population differently. If you have created a rapport of trust and respect with your students, these experiences will be a great learning opportunity for all of you—and can encourage you to try something new. Even better, share the power: Ask the students what adjustments they would make to an activity!

6. There is no "right" answer

As educators, it is natural for us to want to provide young people with the "right" answer. Unfortunately, when talking about something as personal as sex, there often *isn't* one single correct answer. There are many different ways to have "safe sex," many different reasons for engaging in different sexual activity (or not), and many different identities, emotions, and experiences around these topics. Again, within our ethical and pedagogical frameworks, all behaviors that are safe, consensual, and pleasurable are okay. Through your use of games and stories, remember that the more you can stay open to different possibilities, the more your participants will feel in charge of their own bodies and choices.

7. Everything happened, everything is useful

We've all been there: Someone just said something you hadn't anticipated. An activity just took an unexpected turn, and you're not sure how to respond. The important thing to remember in these moments is that they are as much a part of the story as the things you *did* intend to happen. They are there to inform us. When we ignore or avoid things that don't go according to our plan, we deny reality. This can limit our creativity and even lead to shame, when someone feels like their idea or opinion is not valued. Try to be curious about why that person said or did what they did. What might be going on? What is your group trying to tell you? There is no one way to play any of these games, and mistakes are alright—in fact, they are encouraged. Failing in a pretend scenario such as a game actually helps young people build their internal resources and stay resilient in the face of real-life difficulty.

8. Practice saying "yes"

As makers of theatre, we are trained in the art of "**yes, and**." This does not mean going along with any old idea. It means not "blocking." Blocking "is a way of trying to control the situation instead of accepting it. We block when we say no, when we have a better idea, when we change the subject, when we correct the speaker, when we fail to listen, or when we simply ignore the situation."[20] "Saying yes" means affirming any and all experiences—no matter how unsettling, unusual, or unfamiliar. Just as an actor on a stage must "say yes" to the idea that they are Hamlet or Oedipus, a facilitator of participatory theatre can create a space in which learners and leaders are saying "yes" to each other's ideas and experiences.

9. Rehearse for real-life

When we play together in imaginary space, we are rehearsing for real-life experiences. We are scripting moments we might, someday, live out in real-life. Therefore, it is important to do so with the same principles we use for successful interactions in the real world. In that spirit, we offer up this simple, 3-step negotiation framework that will serve you and your learners, both in a theatrical / improvisational context, as well as in your own life experiences:

1. Listen to your partner—Willingly!
2. Express what you want—Clearly!
3. Accept "no"—Gracefully!

Interruption Tactics

As a facilitator in a sexuality education context, you may encounter oppressive, negative, or shaming messages from young people or adults. These kinds of negative comments can throw us off, trigger us, and, if we aren't careful, we can all too easily respond with shame or aggression in return. It is important to be prepared for these kinds of situations. Over time, we have discovered a number of ways to form a positive response to a negative message. A positive response is one that interrupts the negative message and promotes acceptance of multiple perspectives.

The types of responses we have listed below can be used by you, the facilitator, but they can also be used when "in role," or speaking from the perspective of a character. We have found it useful to share these tactics with groups (youth and adults) when we are facilitating, as it provides them with some options for how to respond in a productive way within a game or story structure.

- Asking a question
  - "Can you tell me more about why you feel that way about queer people?"
- Using we-centered language
  - "There are a lot of us who have a different perspective on that, so..."
- Humor
  - "Wait, you said that everyone is having sex all the time? Does that mean I'm having sex right now!?"
- Explaining an emotional response you have
  - "It hurts me to hear that because . . ." "That impacts me because . . ."
- Holding them accountable to their own identity
  - "As a parent, I bet you want your child to be healthy . . ."
  - "As a member of this community, we've agreed to safer space guidelines . . ."
  - "As a teacher, I'm sure you want your students to have all the facts . . ."
- Using facts / data
  - "I can see how you might think that, but that actually isn't true. I read that . . ."
- Using direct language
  - "That's not okay."
  - "That message is oppressive to X community because . . ."
- Personalizing
  - "You know, my brother is actually a survivor of sexual violence, so it makes me really uncomfortable to hear you talking about it in that way."

Sometimes we are asked what "counts" as a negative or "oppressive" message. Simply speaking, an oppressive message is any idea that purports that one group is somehow better than another, and in some measure has the right to control the other group. As you develop your own community guidelines and values, your group might also decide together what feels out of line with those values.

ACTIVITY INDEX

1. BUILD COMMUNITY

Use these game-based activities to cultivate a sense of community and trust within your group.

Activity Name	Description	Content Tag	Level of Exposure
1-1 Yes	Play through verbal and non-verbal modes of giving consent.	#DoesThatCount #MeWe	Low
1-2 Four Corners	Answer open-ended questions, and explore similarities and differences within the group.	#MeWe #StartTheConvo	Low
1-3 The Winds of Change	Find common ground among players.	#StartTheConvo #MeWe	Low
1-4 Affinity Groups	Practice building smaller communities within a larger group.	#BiggerThanUs #MeWe	Low
1-5 Sound and Gesture	Share emotions and ideas about gender through abstract sound and movement.	#MeWe #StartTheConvo	Medium
1-6 Sexy Word Association	Alleviate awkwardness and create shared vocabulary.	#Health411 #StartTheConvo	Medium
1-7 Sociogram	Explore the initial connections between group members.	#StartTheConvo #MeWe	Medium
1-8 That's Awesome	Generate sex-positive ideas with speed and energy.	#Health411 #StartTheConvo	Medium

2. SHARE A STORY

Use these writing and storytelling activities to generate material or reflect on existing material.

Activity Name	Description	Content Tag	Level of Exposure
2-1 Traveling Through Time	Imagine change in a community through writing.	#BiggerThanUs #TakeAction	Low
2-2 Story Fire	Explore & share personal identity through storytelling.	#StartTheConvo #MeWe	Low
2-3 Break Up Letters to Sexual Violence	Identify systemic causes of sexual violence and their symptoms.	#BiggerThanUs #DoesThatCount	Low
2-4 Sex Ed Scripts	Envision learning spaces that meet our needs.	#Health411 #StartTheConvo	Low
2-5 Story Scavenger Hunt	Find themes and patterns among personal stories.	#Health411 #MeWe	Medium
2-6 Affinity Group Story Weaving	Build conceptual links between personal stories.	#MeWe #StartTheConvo	Medium
2-7 Safe-Space Storytelling	Describe elements of safe space through collective storytelling.	#BiggerThanUs #TakeAction	Medium
2-8 Memory Timeline	Recall stories by charting a history of words associated with sex.	#Health411 #StartTheConvo	Medium
2-9 Contraception Speaks	Deepen understanding of and personalize contraception methods.	#Health411 #StartTheConvo	Medium

2-10 Media Messages	Examine and animate media messages about sexuality.	#DoesThatCount #TakeAction	Medium
2-11 Comic Puberty	Draw pictures and write messages to describe puberty experiences.	#Health411 #MeWe	High
2-12 Spectrum of Sexual Behaviors	Examine a range of sexual behaviors as they relate to personal boundaries.	#Health411 #StartTheConvo	High
2-13 Circle of Possibility	Use your imagination to reflect on a successful conversation about your sexual health.	#StartTheConvo	Medium

3. MOVE YOUR BODY
Use these physical activities to get participants out of their heads and moving into action.

Activity Name	Description	Content Tag	Level of Exposure
3-1 Safe Space Tour	Imagine safer spaces through action and reflection.	#BiggerThanUs #TakeAction	Low
3-2 Seated Power	Examine power in relationships by using chairs and body images.	#DoesThatCount #StartTheConvo	Medium
3-3 The First Time I ...	Explore "first" experiences through anonymous storytelling and gesture.	#MeWe, #StartTheConvo	Medium
3-4 Share Your Strategy	Create and emulate gestures for being an ally.	#MeWe #TakeAction	Medium

3-5 I Am a Condom	Explore various settings for conversations about sexual decision-making.	#DoesThatCount #StartTheConvo	Medium
3-6 Relationship Statues	Examine body language and power through still images.	#DoesThatCount #StartTheConvo	Medium
3-7 Maximize/ Minimize	Use still images to explore and express emotional experiences.	#DoesThatCount #StartTheConvo	Medium
3-8 Partnered Power	Investigate power through mirroring.	#DoesThatCount #MeWe	High
3-9 Power Shift	Create images/dialogue that explore power.	#DoesThatCount #MeWe	High
3-10 3-2-1 Anatomy!	Assess knowledge of anatomy through 3-person images.	#Health411	High
3-11 Moving Identities	Embody and explore various identities and the ways they intersect.	#MeWe #StartTheConvo	High
3-12 Can We Touch You?	Practice asking for and responding to physical consent.	#DoesThatCount #MeWe	High

4. ACT IT OUT

Use these role-play activities to help participants explore multiple perspectives and practice for real life scenarios.

Activity Name	Description	Content Tag	Level of Exposure
4-1 Connect and Protect	Interview STI protection methods to choose the right one for different people and contexts.	#Health411	Low

4-2 Myth Busting	Respond to STI-related myths through dialogue and role-play.	#Health411	Medium
4-3 Transforming Oppressive Messages	Play out various interruption strategies to stop oppressive language and behavior.	#StartTheConvo #TakeAction	Medium
4-4 Chance Conflicts	Role-play difficult conversations using group-generated quotes.	#MeWe #TakeAction	Medium
4-5 Sexual Scripts	Break down popular scripts by speaking in cliché.	#DoesThatCount #TakeAction	High
4-6 Make a Choice	Model effective decision-making by playing out multiple approaches to a scenario.	#StartTheConvo #TakeAction	High
4-7 Obstacles in the Road	Practice overcoming challenges to important actions.	#BiggerThanUs #TakeAction	High
4-8 Hack the Circle Game	Play out scenes in role to solve complex problems or situations.	#BiggerThanUs #TakeAction	High

CHAPTER 1: BUILD COMMUNITY

Community is where we begin. Not much that is honest or transformative can happen in a room that feels unwelcoming, unsafe, or unfamiliar. Often at the start of a process, participants will feel uncertain about whether they will find compassion and support for their questions and beliefs from other individuals in the group. By utilizing community-building activities, the facilitator helps to create a safe space rooted in curiosity and respect.

When the facilitator attends to this community from the start, participants will follow suit and maintain it. Instead of shutting others down, they will build upon each others' ideas; instead of jeering at or competing with one another, they will support the group through difficult topics and conversations. Talking about sex can involve a lot of "hard stuff." A strong sense of community will support you through it.

> The game "Yes" is one of the most challenging games in this chapter, and one of my favorites. I remember a residency where this game crashed and burned in one of the first sessions. The group was at this point resistant to working on their feet, and impatient with the grueling repetition of getting this game "right." I encouraged the group to stay with it, and re-introduced the game in future sessions. I hoped the efforts would pay off with a satisfying, empowering breakthrough. But it continued to fall flat.
>
> On our second to last day, I walked in, and I saw that a circle had already begun to form on one side of the room. I assumed at first that it was a circle for chatting, for hanging out. But then I looked closer. A circle of 8 or so students were making eye contact, focusing, and crossing their circle one at a time. They were playing "Yes."
>
> Participatory theatre games bring along their own set of challenges and their own brand of fun. In a game like "Yes," there are no winners or losers. The gratification is not entirely immediate. But in the sometimes messy process, the group forges community, builds trust, and finds a love for the game. Say "Yes" to the activities in this chapter, and enjoy the process (and surprises!) of building community with your participants.
> -   Abby Zan

1-1

YES: PRACTICE VERBAL AND NON-VERBAL MODES OF GIVING CONSENT.

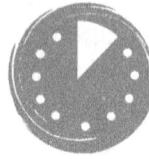

Does That Count

Me We

Preparation: Open space to move

Steps

1. Have the participants form a standing circle.

2. Designate one person to start the game as the Seeker. To begin the **game**, the Seeker will try to find a new place in the circle. To do so, the Seeker will point to another player and say their name out loud.

3. After this Player says "yes," the Seeker can walk toward their new place in the circle. The Player who gave consent is now the Seeker, and must find a new spot.

4. To find a new spot, the new Seeker must point to another player, say their name, and wait for a "Yes."

5. Repeat until the participants are ready for added challenges, reminding the players that they cannot move until they get consent.

6. As the participants get more comfortable, weave in the following challenges:
   - Seekers can no longer speak/ say names, only point.
   - Players must give consent non-verbally.
   - Seekers can no longer point or speak.
   - Players may not use any gestures.

Application

This game is a great warm-up for discussions on healthy communication for any topic (parent/child communication, doctor/patient communication, friends/peer pressure communication, etc.), as well as a way to introduce the concept of consent.

Reflection Questions

- When was it easiest to give consent? To understand if you'd gotten it or not?
- When was it hardest to give/receive consent?
- What does this game teach us about communication?

Notes

This game flows best when students agree to always give consent, and work together to get in tune with each other. We recommend telling participants before gameplay that the game will begin with all "yes" responses, as a way to learn the rules. It's also possible (and more like real consent) to play a variation where players have the option of saying "no" or "yes." If a Player tells a Seeker "No," the Seeker must continue asking Players to leave their spot until they receive a "yes."

This game often needs lots of repetition, and may be used to build trust and ensemble over time.

1-2

FOUR CORNERS:

ANSWER OPEN-ENDED
QUESTIONS & EXPLORE
SIMILARITIES AND DIFFERENCES
WITHIN THE GROUP.

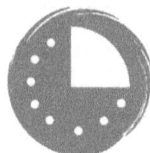

Start The Convo

#Me We

Preparation: List of prompts, open space to move
Connections: Four Corners icebreaker game (origins unknown)

Steps

7. Explain to the participants that for this activity, the walls or corners of the room will be designated as responses to various prompts. When they hear the word "Go," they should move to the spot that best matches their answer.

8. Play through a practice round with only 2 choices. Designate one wall as "choice A" and the other as "choice B." When you say "Go," students will move to the wall that matches their answer. One example could be: Staying up late versus getting up early.

9. Then, introduce all 4 walls as different choices. Some potential prompts could be:
    a. It's easiest to talk about sex with my guardians/my friends/my partner/my doctor.
    b. I'm very comfortable/sort of comfortable/uncomfortable/very uncomfortable talking about sex.
    c. When I'm confused about sex, I typically ask questions to multiple people/I keep quiet about those questions/I ask a trusted friend/I look my question up online.

10. Pause the game periodically to ask participants to share why they are standing where they are standing.

Application

This activity works well as a group get-to-know-you game or to reflect on previously learned content.

Reflection Questions

- Why did you choose this wall?
- Who chose this spot for the same reason?
- Did anyone choose it for a different reason?
- What have we learned about our group today? What should we know if we're going to talk about sex together?

Notes

It may be helpful to ease into the activity with fun and lower-exposure prompts (favorite foods, TV shows, school subjects, etc.)

Some students may have difficulty choosing—this is ok! Designate a spot in the room for "don't know," or allow the room to function more like a spectrum (i.e. it's ok to stand between two choices).

1-3

THE WINDS OF CHANGE: FIND COMMON
GROUND BETWEEN PLAYERS.

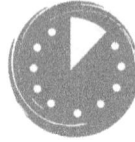

Start The Convo

Me We

Preparation: Circle of chairs
Connection: The icebreaker "A Big Wind Blows" (origin unknown)

Steps

1. The participants form a seated circle in chairs. The facilitator stands in the center of the circle to demonstrate game-play (the following structure assumes that facilitators will also play!).

2. The game begins when the player in the middle shares one true thing about themselves that is not immediately visible.

3. Everyone for whom this statement is also true must stand up and find a new seat. Like musical chairs, someone will be left standing. They will then stand in the middle of the circle to share a new fact about themselves.

4. Remind players to use statements that don't relate to appearance. The goal of the game is to learn things about each other that we couldn't tell just by looking at one another. Examples of prompts we've used include: Has older siblings, city of origin, favorite snack, etc.

5. Play the game through several rounds until all interested players have had a chance in the middle.

Application

This game is useful for finding common ground between diverse groups of players and can lead to discussions around identity. It can also be applied within a theme like family-centered facts, facts from childhood, or dreams for the future.

Reflection Questions

- After playing this game, what do we know about us as a group?
- Were you surprised by any of the similarities you found with others?

Notes

Sometimes participants, especially younger folks, may resist going in the middle. To reduce the risk of being "the only one," you can add the rule: If something is true only for the speaker, everyone resets by yelling YOU'RE UNIQUE! and moving to a new seat.

1-4

AFFINITY GROUPS:
PRACTICE BUILDING SMALLER COMMUNITIES WITHIN A LARGER GROUP.

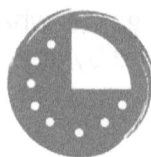

◎ **Bigger Than Us**

◉ **Me We**

Preparation: Open space to move

Steps

1. Invite participants to walk around the room and cover the space.

2. As participants practice walking around the room, remind them to use soft focus—using their front and peripheral vision, as well as all their senses—to be aware of the people in the room.

3. Begin to share prompts from the list. When the players hear the word "Go!" they will silently form affinity groups—groups that share like traits based on the prompts. Begin with something simple such as "type of footwear."

4. On the count of 3, ask each member of the affinity group to name their group at the same time, with no discussion beforehand. Notice any differences in how members name their group. Repeat this for each existing group.

5. Repeat with various prompts such as age, height, hairstyle, and clothing.

6. For an added challenge, use prompts that are less outwardly apparent such as favorite season, mood today, favorite extracurricular activity, hopes for the future, etc.

Application

This game can be used to build community and discuss shared identities. It can also be used to discuss invisible identities and stereotypes.

Equally important, it can be used to discuss successful improvisation skills like "**Yes, and**" and eye contact.

Reflection Questions

- What made this game hard? What made it easier?
- What did this game teach us about our group? What do we have in common? What differentiates us?
- What skills did we practice in this game? How might these skills help us in discussing/learning about sex and sexuality?

Notes

The biggest challenge in this game is staying silent while forming and naming groups. Explain that this rule helps challenge us to find new ways to collaborate and communicate.

Sample Facilitation Script

(Note: We like to facilitate this and other cover-the-space activities while walking or moving around the room alongside participants.)

FACILITATOR: *Begin to move around the room. Find a nice, medium pace that's comfortable for you. Cover as much space as you can. Notice where your eyes are looking—at other people in the room? At the walls or the floor? Let's move into a type of vision called "soft focus." Look straight ahead of you and relax your eyes. Without moving your eyes, try to see as much of the room as you can at one time—in front of you, left, and right. Hold on to this soft focus for the rest of the game, so you can look where you're going and see as much of the room as possible. For this game, we will keep moving around the room and using our awareness.*

As we walk I'll call out a category—something you should be able to see on other people in the room. Then without talking, we'll put ourselves into groups based on the word I call out. The first category is FOOTWEAR. Look for others in the room wearing something similar on their feet, and create a group. Make sure you spread out so it's clear which group is which.

(Give the room a few minutes to sort themselves into groups)

Now, freeze wherever you are! Without talking to your other group members, look around and decide what you think the name of your group is based on your footwear. When I point to your group, on the count of three, shout out this name. It's okay if you say different words—that's part of the fun.

(Point to each group one by one, countdown, "*3, 2, 1, Go.*")

Let's start to cover the space again. Return to your soft focus, and your awareness of all the other bodies and objects in the room. In a moment, I'll say a category again. Just like last time, we'll put ourselves into groups without talking. The category is . . .

(Continue to play through a few more categories, making them as challenging as you'd like! If you are moving into a group-based activity after this one, you can try using the final round of the game to land in those groups.)

Side coaching pointers:

- *If you're moving around in the same circle over and over again, switch it up!*

- *Be aware of where others are in the room. Are you using all of your senses to take in the space?*
- *Working together without talking is the most challenging part of this game. What are some other ways to communicate? How can you use your body to express yourself?*

1-5

SOUND & GESTURE: SHARE
FEELINGS AND IDEAS ABOUT
GENDER THROUGH ABSTRACT
SOUND AND MOVEMENT.

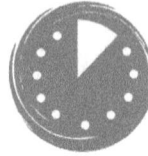

Start The Convo

Me We

Preparation: Open space to move

Steps

1. Have the participants form a standing circle.

2. Explain that each participant will perform a sound and gesture that shares something about their **gender** in this moment. Remind participants to avoid words. After each person goes, the entire group will repeat back their sound and gesture.

3. Demonstrate your current personal gender through sound and gesture first. Examples we have seen include putting on lipstick, posing like a superhero, and examples that flip binaries on the head. Wait for the group to perform it back.

4. Go around the circle, with each participant sharing their sound/gesture, and the group repeating it back.

5. After one complete circle, the group performs the same sound and gestures in half the time to build energy.

Application

This activity can be modified for many uses and topics:
*   A group introduction game: Perform the sound and gesture that tell the group something about you.
*   A group thermometer: Create a gesture that indicates how you are feeling in that moment, share something you love or something you are, etc.

Reflection Questions

- What is the difference between **gender identity** and **gender expression**?
- How can gender expression vary, even among those who share the same gender identity?
- Where have we seen these gestures before?
- How did it feel to perform other people's gestures?

Notes

Participants may need to take some time to define **gender** (see glossary). Remind participants that gender is fluid and can change in the moment. This game provides a good way to tune into gender nuance.

Depending on age, responses may lean heavily into stereotypes. This is useful! Take the time to question where we have seen these sounds/gestures before or what it felt like to repeat these gestures (especially across genders).

1-6

SEXY WORD ASSOCIATION:
ALLEVIATE AWKWARDNESS AND CREATE SHARED VOCABULARY.

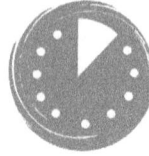

Start The Convo

Health 411

Preparation: Open space to move
Connections: Improvisational Theatre

Steps

1. As a warm-up, have the participants form a standing circle, and make a slow and steady beat using light snaps or claps.

2. Pause the group rhythm to provide instructions, and choose someone to start the **game**.

3. The game play begins when one player says a word they associate with sex (e.g. "pleasure"), on the beat.

4. The player to their left will then say the first word they think of in response, like "chest," on the next beat.

5. After those two words are said, the full group will combine both words into one phrase on the next beat, and say "pleasure chest."

6. On the next and final beat, everyone says, 'You got it!'"

7. A sample turn sounds like this:
    a. *Participant 1: Pleasure*
    b. *Participant 2: Chest*
    c. *All: Pleasure Chest*
    d. *All: You got it!*

8. After one player responds to the previous player's word, they offer a new word to the person on their left. This process continues on the beat until each participant gets a chance to respond to a word and offer their own.

Application

Use this activity to break through awkwardness and get participants laughing. It's also extremely helpful when assessing what sexuality-related vocabulary a group already uses.

Reflection Questions

- What made this game easy? What made it hard?
- Did we notice any patterns in the kinds of words that came up?

Notes

The point is not to string together two words that necessarily match or make a coherent phrase. Even nonsense words work! Whatever comes to mind first should be said and accepted.

To avoid getting stuck trying to think of clever words, remind participants to focus foremost on keeping the beat. If you want, you could offer a list of words to work from initially, perhaps using a vocabulary list.

If the group catches on quickly, play with speeding up the tempo!

1-7

SOCIOGRAM: Explore
THE INITIAL CONNECTIONS BETWEEN GROUP MEMBERS.

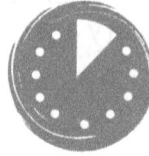

Start The Convo

Me We

Preparation: List of prompts, open space to move

Steps

1. Invite the participants to walk around the room and **cover the space**.

2. As participants practice walking around the room, remind them to use **soft focus**—using their front and peripheral vision, as well as all their senses—to be aware of the people in the room.

3. The game play begins when a prompt is shared. Players will then place their hand on the shoulder of someone according to the prompt and freeze.

4. Between each prompt, give the participants time to walk around the space and re-set.

5. Prompts should activate interest and inquiry in our identities, both seen and unseen. Prompts can include:
   a. Someone who you think is very similar to you
   b. Someone who you think is very different from you
   c. Someone who you think is a good ally
   d. Someone who you would feel comfortable going to with a question about your sexual health
   e. Someone who you would trust to rescue you in the middle of the night from a dangerous place
   f. Someone who you wish you knew more about

6. Participants can choose to abstain from any of the prompts by freezing with their hands at their sides.

Application

This activity gives participants a nonverbal way to explore their initial feelings and assumptions about others in the group.

Reflection Questions

- Why did you make the choices you did?
- Which choices were easy to make? Which were harder? Why?
- Was anyone surprised at being selected?
- Questions can be given between prompts or at the end of the game.

Notes

In order to ensure everyone chosen feels complimented and not put down, keep all prompts positive.

In some groups, especially with shy students or participants who do not yet know each other, choosing a person for each prompt may be difficult. Some of us have found success designating a spot to stand that means "I don't know." This is most effective when coupled with reflection: Why did so many of us have trouble choosing someone for X prompt? How do we demonstrate that we are worthy of this trust?

1-8

THAT'S AWESOME:
GENERATE SEX-POSITIVE IDEAS
WITH SPEED AND ENERGY.

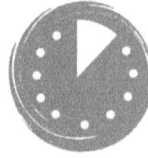

Start The Convo

Health 411

Preparation: Open space to move
Connections: Improvisational Theatre

Steps

1. Have the participants form a standing circle.

2. The game play begins when you call out a player's name and ask them to give you "3 Reasons" for various **sex-positive** prompts. The focus of this **game** should be on speaking quickly, without thought, rather than coming up with something clever. Even nonsense words or sounds are ok!

3. After each reason listed, the group shouts "1!" then "2!" then "3!" After "3!" the group shouts, "That's awesome!"

4. A sample turn looks like this:
   Facilitator: Rachel, give me 3 reasons why you love yourself
   Student 1: Because I'm awesome!
   All: 1!
   Student 1: Because I'm cool as a cucumber!
   All: 2!
   Student 1: Because when I play the piano, I'm on fire!
   All: 3! That's awesome!

5. Continue around the circle, giving each person a chance to respond to a prompt. Prompts may include:
   a. Reasons why you can be yourself
   b. Reasons why sex can be good
   c. Reasons why it's okay to say no
   d. Reasons why it's great to be gay
   e. Reasons why someone would use an internal condom
   f. Reasons why someone would use hormonal contraception
   g. Reasons why someone might not use contraception

Application

This is a playful way to mine for ideas that support positive, healthy sexual behaviors. It also helps participants practice expressing and defending their views and values to others. Apply this activity to any content area that you want to draw positivity towards.

Reflection Questions

- What made this game hard? What made it easy?

Notes

This game is most successful when played fast. Encourage the participant who is generating responses not to get in their head. They should say the first thing that comes to mind, even if it is complete nonsense.

CHAPTER 2: SHARE A STORY

As educators, stories can help us bring personal relevance to abstract information and ideas. They help us to forge meaningful connections with others around important topics. In particular, sharing stories about sex and sexuality can help young people feel a little less alone in the world. Stories help young people realize that others might understand where they are coming from, might have been in their shoes before, and might even have an idea about how they can move forward.

Unfortunately, the narrative often told about teenagers, especially in mainstream media, is largely one-note, not to mention unfair: Young people are lazy, they're rude, and they're self-involved. In a health context, the stories are even less empathetic: Young people are irresponsible, they don't take anything seriously, and they don't know what's best for them.

We need new stories of young people's health. We need to make space for young people to tell their own stories. Speaking our stories aloud is like speaking ourselves into existence: We express our fears, joys, frustrations, and dreams, and hope that they resonate with our community at large. Sharing stories can help young people and adults dream a better world—and more empowering narratives of adolescent sexual health—into reality.

One afternoon I was talking with a group of high school students about power in relationships. We made a list of things that can give people power (money, age, size, gender, race, being "less in-love," knowing a secret, etc.). Our conversation turned to equal power. What did that look like? How could we create it in our relationships? Here, we hit a roadblock. One young woman raised her hand and said, "I'm sorry but sometimes it just is. Sometimes people just don't treat each other like equals." Other students agreed. They had seen plenty of relationships where one person held more power. It was normal. Shared power was corny and unattainable.

We decided to write down, in groups, the beginning of a story about a relationship that was unequal. Students wrote about couples where the man always paid for everything, parent-child relationships where parents took away phones, peer-to-peer interactions where bigger kids got the best seats. Students then wrote a "happy ending" version of the story, where the inequality went away. Once we had a beginning and an end, students took the time to figure out the "middle" of the story. What actions or conversations moved the relationship from unequal to equal?

Although students may have lacked models of realistic, positive relationships in their own lives, they were able to create these kinds of relationships in the stories they wrote. Storytelling allowed us to bypass a roadblock of perceived reality, delve deep into conversation, and imagine new paths to fostering healthy, power-sharing models of relationships.
-   Shannon Oliver-O'Neil

2-1

TRAVELING THROUGH TIME:

IMAGINE CHANGE IN A
COMMUNITY THROUGH WRITING.

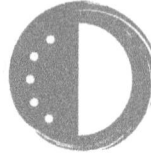

Bigger Than Us

Take Action

Preparation: Writing materials, seated writing area

Steps

1. Ask the participants to think of one community they belong to, and one way they would like it to be different. Tell them to write that change down, as if it already happened. For example: The school began offering comprehensive sex ed to every student.

2. Participants should then travel backward and imagine what happened just before the change occurred by writing 10 consecutive sentences that begin with "Before that . . .". For example: Before that, students formed a coalition with teachers to advocate for better sex ed.

3. Remind writers that sentences should be action-oriented (what happened?) rather than descriptive (how did it feel)?

4. Participants will then travel forward and imagine what happened just after the change occurred by writing 10 consecutive sentences that begin with, 'Because of that . . .'". For example: Because of that, students learned about their options for contraception at school.

5. As before, the sentences should be action-oriented rather than descriptive.

6. The participants then share out important sentences from their stories **popcorn-style**, or all at once, depending on their comfort level.

Application

Use this activity to develop concrete action plans around a change that your group is working to achieve, or use it to think idealistically and imaginatively.

Reflection Questions

- What part of this activity was hard? Why? What was easy? Why?
- What can we take away from what we heard?
- Did this feel realistic? Why or why not?

Notes

If writing abilities vary within the group, or silent work is hard, it may be useful to place students in pairs with one storyteller and one scribe.

THE SEX ED PLAYBOOK

2-2

STORY FIRE: EXPLORE AND SHARE PERSONAL IDENTITY THROUGH STORYTELLING.

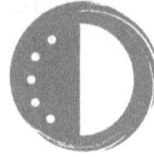

Health 411

Me We

Preparation: Writing materials, open space to move and write

Steps

1. Ask the participants to write a 3-line story about sexual identity, either personal or witnessed (remind participants to be mindful of folks' privacy if telling a story that involves other people!).

2. Participants speak their story aloud quietly to themselves, until they've memorized all three lines. For example: My friend and I went to the mall. / He came out to me in the food court as we shared a plate of fries. / I told him I'd always have his back.

3. Participants **cover the space**, using **soft focus**, until the facilitator cues them to stop and find a partner. Participants share their stories with their partner. Participants choose one line from their partner's story to replace a line in their own story. Then, they continue to move around the room until they are instructed to stop and find a new partner. With each new story, they must replace one sentence of their story with someone else's. For example: My friend and I went to the mall. / I'm still trying to figure out who I am. / I told him I'd always have his back.

4. After 2 to 3 minutes of sharing and transforming stories, the facilitator selects participants to speak the final version of the story they developed throughout the game.

Application

This activity applies the concept of story scavenger hunts to sexual identity. However, facilitators can substitute any core concept that youth might have personal stories around.

Reflection Questions

- Which themes emerged?
- How did you decide which sentences to incorporate into your story?

Notes

You may offer more structure for the initial story prompt, according to your objectives and your group. For example, choose a story about a moment of identity discovery, sharing that identity with someone else, celebrating that identity, etc.

If participants have trouble with memorization, encourage them to jot down their story and the new lines they adapt.

2-3

BREAK-UP LETTERS TO SEXUAL VIOLENCE: IDENTIFY SYSTEMIC CAUSES OF SEXUAL VIOLENCE AND THEIR SYMPTOMS.

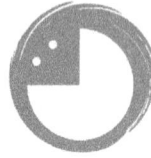

Bigger Than Us

Does That Count

Preparation: Writing materials, seated writing areas

Steps

1. Ask the participants to write letters breaking up with **sexual violence**. Have the participants start with "Dear Sexual Violence" at the top, and list all of the qualities of the culture that aren't working out for them. The letters may finish with the participant's plans for moving on.

2. Have the participants read aloud sentences or phrases that stand out to them, **popcorn style**.

Application

Writing break up letters can be a powerful tool for ending relationships with anything we don't want to play a part in our lives, like addictions, oppressions, self-doubt, etc.

Reflection Questions

- What resonated for you?
- What surprised you?
- What themes emerged?

Notes

This activity looks at survivor and perpetrator stories not as isolated events but as a part of larger systems that support the existence of sexual violence in our lives. Rather than focusing on any one individual, break-up letters should address the components and culture of sexual violence, like rape myths, victim blaming, not believing survivors, toxic masculinity, etc.

2-4

SEX ED SCRIPTS:

ENVISION LEARNING SPACES
THAT MEET OUR NEEDS.

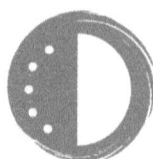

◎ **Health 411**

? **Start The Convo**

Preparation: Writing materials, tables for group work, open space for performance area

Steps

1. In pairs or small groups, have the participants write a script for the first day of the worst sex ed class they can imagine. Invite the participants to write using a teacher and students as characters.

2. Ask for volunteer pairs/groups to share their scenes aloud in the performance area.

3. After the participants have shared their scenes, guide a discussion to pull out the themes about what makes those classes bad (i.e., shaming language, boring, lack of information, etc.).

4. After listing negative approaches, have the participants return to their groups to write the reverse: A list of the top 5 elements of good sexuality education, where they set their own standards. If time allows, the participants may revise and share their first scenes according to these new standards.

Application

Use this activity to elicit ideas about what topics to cover. It is particularly useful to assess the needs of your group at the beginning of a program.

Reflection Questions

- Which scenario was easier to write? Why?
- Did you discover anything new about your values during this activity?

Notes

Allow the participants to work individually or in groups, as best suits the writing skills of the room.

2-5

STORY SCAVENGER HUNT: FIND THEMES AND PATTERNS AMONG PERSONAL STORIES.

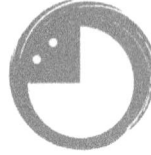

Health 411

Me We

Preparation: Writing materials, a Scavenger Hunt Checklist, seated writing areas, open space to move

Steps

1. Ask the participants to think of an experience they have had surrounding teenage pregnancy, either personal or witnessed. Provide prompts to inspire participant writing, such as:
    a. What myths have you heard about teenage pregnancy? How do your stories bust those myths open?
    b. Where is the joy in the story? Where is the struggle?
    c. Who is the hero in the story?

2. The participants will take 10 minutes to write down their story in 5 or more sentences.

3. When the stories are completed, the facilitator hands each participant a Scavenger Hunt Checklist. This is a list of themes that may be encountered in these stories, such as:
    a. Shame
    b. Strength
    c. Personal Connection
    d. Access to Resources
    e. Lack of Access to Resources
    f. Obstacles

4. Have the participants move into pairs to begin the scavenger hunt. The facilitator may prompt participants to select partners at random as they move through the space (as in Story Fire), or create a Speed-Dating style rotation with chairs.

5. Prompt the pairs to decide who will share first. Then, say "Go!" After 1 to 2 minutes, cue the participants to switch to the second partner. As they listen, participants should check off any items from the Checklist that they hear in their partners' stories.

6. Have the participants continue rotating through different pairs until someone checks off all components on their Scavenger Hunt Checklist.

Application

This activity applies the concept of story scavenger hunts to teenage pregnancy. However, facilitators can substitute any core concept that participants might have personal stories around.

Reflection Questions

- What connections did we notice?
- Which items on our checklist were easiest to find? Which items were hardest? Why do you think that might be?

Notes

The scavenger hunt checklist should list whatever components feel most relevant to the lesson. Be sure to choose prompts that affirm all safe and consensual experiences rather than shame particular choices that a young person might make.

2-6

AFFINITY STORY GROUP WEAVING:
BUILD CONCEPTUAL LINKS BETWEEN PERSONAL STORIES.

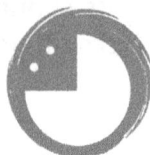

Start The Convo

Me We

Preparation: Writing materials, open space to move

Steps

1. Follow directions for Affinity Group exercise 1-4.

2. After a few rounds of this, ask the participants to find a partner within their **affinity group**.

3. Offer the participants a storytelling prompt inspired by the group theme. For example, if the affinity groups are based on "shoes," the prompt might be, *"Tell a story about a time you walked a mile in somebody's shoes."*

4. Participants choose who will be the Storyteller first, and who will be the Listener. Invite the Listener to listen actively to their partner's story, then write down 1 to 3 quotes from that story afterwards.

5. Storyteller has 1 to 2 minutes to share their story; Listener writes 1 to 3 quotes. Then, have the participants switch roles.

6. Have the partners share quotes with each other, and ask for consent to use each quote in the next activity. The quotes that are not consented to are off limits for future play.

7. Have the group form a standing circle and ask one person to move into the circle.

8. The game play begins when the person in the middle shares a quote from their partner's story. They use the quote as a jumping

off point for telling their partner's story in first person. The Teller should speak continuously until tapped out by another participant.

9. Instruct the participants to tap into the story weaving when they hear a word or concept related to their own partner's quotes. The participants enter the circle by calling out that word or concept. For instance, if a story is shared about moms and another participant has a family-related quote, they can call out "Family," and then tap into the circle.

10. Play through a few rounds, reminding participants that there are no right or wrong interpretations of theme or connections between the stories. Give the participants permission to re-use words and concepts for multiple stories.

Application

This activity can help examine commonalities and differences of identities within groups.

It can also be used to explore and generate content around a theme by seeing what personal connections come up when we limit prompts to a specific content area (e.g. pregnancy, body image, etc.).

Reflection Questions

- What words or concepts came up most often in our story weaving?
- What questions did these stories bring up for you?
- What did it feel like to tell someone else's story/hear someone tell yours?
- How do we take care of one another when handling stories that are not our own?

Notes

Depending on timing & goals, you may play through additional rounds of steps 2-5, generating multiple stories, before moving into story weaving.

2-7

SAFE-SPACE STORYTELLING:
DESCRIBE ELEMENTS OF SAFE SPACE THROUGH COLLECTIVE STORYTELLING.

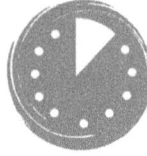

Bigger Than Us

Take Action

Preparation: Open space to move

Steps

1. Have the participants form a seated circle.

2. As a group, brainstorm specific elements that create a **safe space**. Encourage participants to use their senses: *What does this world look/sound/smell like? What do you see there?*

3. Have the participants collectively tell a story about an imagined safe space, and how it came to be that way. The game play begins when one player tells the first sentence of a story, beginning with the words "Once upon a time ..."

4. The participant to their left will tell the next line of the story. Remind participants to keep in mind the principle of **"Yes, and,"** to continue to build upon the same story, rather than contradict what came before.

5. Continue around the circle, with each participant sharing one sentence until the story comes to an end.

6. Participants can end the sentence by saying "Period."

Application

Use this activity to tell a story on any theme, especially if the initial brainstorm involves specific, sensory images for participants to build upon.

With the given prompt, this game can help create shared culture/vocabulary for the group, and provide a jumping off point for discussing group agreements.

Reflection Questions

- What themes came up in our story?
- How might we bring some of the elements of our fictional safe space into the space we share together?

Notes

Some participants may prefer to prepare a list of safe space elements in advance, before sharing in the full group. Use your best judgment as a facilitator for what your group needs.

THE SEX ED PLAYBOOK

2-8

MEMORY TIMELINE: RECALL STORIES BY CHARTING A HISTORY OF WORDS ASSOCIATED WITH SEX.

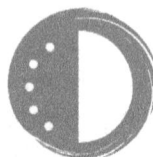

Health 411

Start The Convo

Preparation: Markers, Post-it notes (several for each participant), large paper or board to write on

Steps

1. Create a large, visible timeline with tick marks for all the age ranges in participants' lifetimes, from birth to present age (e.g., ages 1-5, 6-10, 11-15, 16-20, etc.).

2. Prompt the participants to write any words they associated with sex in their lifetime on post-it notes (one word/phrase per post-it).

3. Ask the participants to place their individual words/phrases under the age-range during which they first encountered them.

4. After the timeline is complete, examine the wall as a group. Discuss any themes or reflections.

5. Ask each participant to examine the wall and find a word that reminds them of a story in their own lives. Participants will take the post-it off the wall once they have chosen one.

6. Pair up the participants. Ask the participants to share a story with their partner that's associated with the post-it they chose.

Application

This game can be modified to explore multiple themes by changing the timeline ticks to things like "Experiences of the media," "Terms you used for anatomical parts," or "Educational milestones."

Reflection Questions

- What patterns did we see in our timeline?
- Did you see anything that surprised you?
- Based on the words we put up, what could a stranger guess about our experiences with sex ed?

Notes

Set up some invitations and boundaries about vocabulary at the outset of this exercise. For example, participants often need permission to use words that aren't typically allowed in their classroom setting (e.g. slang).

If you see the same words written over and over, encourage participants to dig deeper with different words—the more variety on the board, the richer the exploration. Be sure to point out repetition when it does happen, which can be an indicator of themes in the group.

2-9

CONTRACEPTION SPEAKS: DEEPEN UNDERSTANDING OF AND PERSONALIZE CONTRACEPTION METHODS.

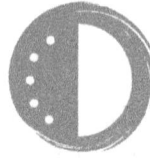

Health 411

Start The Convo

Preparation: Writing materials, contraception cards, seated writing area

Steps

1. Introduce this activity after participants have learned about different methods of **contraception**. Assign each participant a contraception method (e.g., hormonal birth control, abstinence, IUD) by passing them a card with the method written on it. Facilitators may include quick facts about the method on the card, for participants' reference.

2. Instruct the participants to write a monologue from the perspective of their given contraception, explaining personal strengths and struggles. Prompts to guide writing could include:
   a. I hope . . .
   b. I fear . . .
   c. I love . . .
   d. I forget . . .
   e. I believe in . . .

3. Ask the participants to share out important sentences **popcorn-style**, or read their monologues in character, depending on the comfort level of the group.

Application

This activity can be used to playfully explore behavioral, hormonal, or barrier methods of protection. By personifying contraception methods, the participants can become more familiar with the specifics of each method and its advantages/disadvantages.

Reflection Questions

- Which methods did you identify with? Why?
- Which methods did not appeal to you? Why?
- What follow-up questions do you have for the contraception characters you heard from?

Notes

It is helpful to provide cards with accurate information for participants to use when building their characters. Or, you could have them choose a contraception method and research it with trusted online or print resources.

Remind the participants that there are no wrong answers, and it's okay to be silly. Remind them that we are trying to imagine, "What if?" these methods could talk, think, and feel?

2-10

MEDIA MESSAGES:
EXAMINE AND ANIMATE MEDIA
MESSAGES ABOUT SEXUALITY.

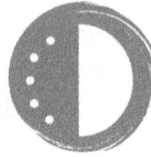

(?) **Does That Count**

(▶) **Take Action**

Preparation: Writing materials, seated writing area, large paper or board to write on

Steps

1. Ask the participants to think of a message from the media or pop culture (a song lyric, line from a movie or show, online article, etc.) that has made them think about their sexuality. Write a few ideas on the board.

2. Then, participants write down additional messages using the exact words that the media source used and/or write from the media's point of view.
   a. (i.e. Instead of writing *"The media told me that I have to be thin to be beautiful,"* participants should write, *"You have to be thin to be beautiful."*)

3. As a group, have the participants share out and reflect on reactions to the messages.

4. Tell the participants to expand on their message with a monologue. Ask them to write about what they would think, do or say if they were someone who believed this message.

Application

This activity can be done by writing messages from sources other than the media (parent/guardian, peers, school, close friends, etc.).

Reflection Questions

- How do these messages make you feel?
- How might they impact the way we think about sex?

- How often do we encounter these messages?
- Do you believe them? Why or why not?

Notes

To activate this game further, participants can play in role as one of the voices from the monologues. Pair one positive messenger with one negative messenger to explore how they might be in conversation together.

If participants are reluctant to share a message/lyric that has directly impacted their own sexuality, the prompt can be broadened to include messages that "people our age" have heard about sexuality.

2-11

PUBERTY COMICS:

DRAW PICTURES AND WRITE
MESSAGES TO DESCRIBE PUBERTY
EXPERIENCES.

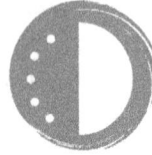

Health 411

Me We

Preparation: Unlined paper and crayons/markers for each participant; tables for group work

Steps

1. Have the participants sit in groups of 4 to 6, and provide each group with a piece of paper and drawing instrument.

2. Ask the participants to tri-fold the paper vertically and label the sections 1 to 6 (1-3 on the front, 4-6 on the back).

3. Ask participants to work in sequence, adding to each other's ideas in the following manner:
   a. On panel 1, in one sentence, describe a change a young person might experience during puberty. Pass the paper to the left.
   b. Look at panel one, then fold it so only panel 2 shows and illustrate this sentence. Pass the paper to the left.
   c. Look at panel 2, then fold it so only panel 3 shows. Write an inner thought or a mantra that a young person could say to inspire pride about the illustrated change. Pass the paper to the left.
   d. Look at panel 3, then fold it so only panel 4 shows. Illustrate this inner thought or mantra. Pass the paper to the left.
   e. Look at panel 4, then fold it so only panel 5 shows. Write a message a young person could share with another young person to help them feel like the picture. Pass the paper to the left.
   f. Fold the paper so only panel 6 shows. Illustrate this message.

4. Ask each group to share their Puberty Comics.

Application

This type of collaborative drawing and writing activity can be used to tackle any health content by switching out the drawing and writing prompts.

Reflection Questions

- What do these comics tell us about how young people may experience puberty?
- What obstacles did we see the comic characters encounter?
- What powers or sources of strength did we see?

Notes

Use newly generated comic strips as inspiration for scene work and future play.
This activity draws on the concept of Exquisite Corpse, a surrealist drawing game.

2-12

SPECTRUM OF SEXUAL BEHAVIORS: EXAMINE A RANGE OF SEXUAL BEHAVIORS AS THEY RELATE TO PERSONAL BOUNDARIES.

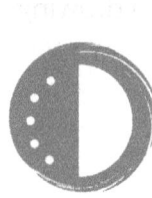

Health 411

Start The Convo

Preparation: Game surface (board or paper containing spectrum with "Most Comfortable" on one end and "Least Comfortable" on the other), Behavior Cards (7-10 smaller slips of paper containing sexual behaviors on them, like going on a date with friends, oral sex, sending/receiving nude pictures, etc.), writing materials

Steps

1. A facilitator will pass out one game board (or worksheet), and one set of behavior cards to each participant.

2. The game play begins when participants place behavior cards along the spectrum to create their personal comfort spectrum. Participants can leave out any cards they don't want to use, for whatever reason.

3. Ask the group to imagine that they or another person they know identified one of these behaviors as "off limits."

4. Tell participants to write 5 different ways to respond to someone asking them to engage in that activity. All responses should respect their "No."

5. Share out and reflect as a group.

Application

This activity can be used to assess comfort for any kind of risky behavior or any behavior that demands boundary-setting.

Reflection Questions

- Did our responses feel realistic? Why or why not?
- Was it easy to sort the behavior cards in the game? Why or why not?
- How do we think our game boards might look different over the course of our lives?

Notes

Sexual behaviors for each game card can also be sourced from/created by the group ahead of time.

2-13

CIRCLE OF POSSIBILITY: USE YOUR IMAGINATION TO REFLECT ON A SUCCESSFUL CONVERSATION ABOUT YOUR SEXUAL HEALTH.

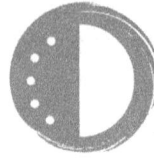

Start The Convo

Preparation: Chairs for participation
Connections: Devising Structures

Steps

1. The facilitator organizes the participants in pairs. Have the participants sit in chairs facing each other.

2. Ask the participants to imagine they just had a breakthrough conversation about their sexual health with someone important to them (a partner, parent, doctor, etc.). This conversation can be entirely fictional or one they have already had.

3. Ask the participants to share with their partner what happened and why the conversation was so successful. Remind participants that anything is possible and to speak as if the event has already occurred, if imaginary.

4. Explain that those who are listening to the story should ask questions that add detail or complexity to the story, as if they had been there, too: "*And then your doctor gave you free condoms, right?*" or "*And your mom was totally cool about your boyfriend?*" The Storyteller should practice **"Yes, and,"** and incorporate as many of the Listeners' ideas into their story as they like.

5. Demonstrate the activity with a volunteer before the groups begin. Show the participants how to speak about an imagined conversation and how to ask good, probing questions.

6. Debrief the activity by sharing any highlights or discoveries. Then, brainstorm what would need to happen in order to make this sort of conversation possible, or what was in place for successful conversations that already happened, and identify action steps participants might take to get there.

Application

This activity allows participants a safety net to say or imagine something that they might not believe is actually possible, along with naming positive conversations that have already happened. It also plants the seeds for positive conversation strategies and possible discoveries about how to structure productive dialogue in the future.

Reflection Questions

- What surprised you about the situation you described?
- What tools did you gain to use in future conversations?

Sample Facilitation Script

(NOTE: Prior to starting the activity, organize students in partners or small groups. Have them sit in chairs facing each other.)

FACILITATOR: *In this activity, we are going to imagine what successful conversations about sexual health look like. We'll start by imagining our own version of this quietly to ourselves. You're welcome to think of a conversation you have actually had before (if that's safe to talk about in this room) or to imagine one that hasn't taken place yet. So take a minute now to imagine what a successful conversation about sexual health looks like for you. It may help to look down or close your eyes. Who are you having this conversation with: Your friend? Your partner? Your doctor? A family member? Imagine the setting: Where does it happen? How does the setting help make the conversation a positive one? And what is this conversation about? What kinds of questions are you or the other person asking? How do you imagine you would feel before this conversation? During? After? Take another minute on your own to think through any other details I might not have asked about.*

Now, we're going to interview our partners about these imaginary conversations. Can I get a volunteer who feels comfortable being interviewed in front of the group?

(Find a volunteer, and have them sit across from you to model the interview.)

FACILITATOR: *So first, my partner is going to share with me what happened briefly. My role as your partner is going to be to listen well. Once you've told me a little about the conversation, I'll ask questions that help draw out the details. As your partner, I'm going to try to practice "Yes, and," and ask questions that help continue to develop this story. Let's try it.*

(The volunteer shares their story. The facilitator engages them by asking follow up questions in a conversational manner. For example, *"So you had this whole conversation in the waiting room before your appointment? Did you worry that people would overhear you? How did you feel afterward? And then the doctor gave you condoms, right? Where did you put them?"*)

(After a few minutes of play, the facilitator should pause the game, and get a suggestion or two from the group for other probing questions you

THE SEX ED PLAYBOOK

could ask this volunteer. Use this as an opportunity to point out great examples of "**Yes, and**," and/or name the places where improvisers can improve.)

FACILITATOR: *Thanks so much, (volunteer)! Now, everyone turn to your partner(s), and decide who is going to share first. First storytellers, start telling your story.*

(Give the first storytellers 5 to 10 minutes to share and respond to questions; then have them switch partners. Once the conversations have wrapped up, instruct the group to form a circle with their chairs. Lead a reflection and brainstorm that best suits your group's needs.)

Sample Reflection and Brainstorm Prompts:

- *What made the conversations in your stories successful?*
- *Did any challenges or surprises come up in your conversations? If so, did your group members/partners have ideas for how to address them?*
- *What would it take to make these conversations happen in real life? Can we brainstorm some actions to make these conversations possible?* (These ideas could be written down on a board or other shared space; or, this could turn into an individual journaling activity.)

CHAPTER 3 - MOVE YOUR BODY

Too much time in our nation's classrooms is spent sitting at desks, facing a whiteboard or a teacher at the front of a room. As educators, we are generally comfortable with this setup: We can tell students are listening to us if they are looking at us and sitting still. There are certainly situations—particularly ones that involve memorization or individual work—for which this setup makes sense as a way to learn. However, this is *one way* to learn. What happens when everyone gets out of their seats? How does an educator host a space where students are making connections and processing in new, "on-our-feet" ways?

> *I arrived at a Chicago middle school to co-facilitate a professional development workshop for teachers on how to positively respond to students with questions about sexual health topics. The teachers filed into the room, sitting at separate tables with plates of snacks, and looking down at their phones or handouts. When we began they were engaged, politely interested, but still sitting back. I asked that they move their chairs and tables to the sides of the room to stand up for a game. It was like they were moving in slow motion. The resistance to getting up on their feet was clear.*

> *Once in a circle, I gave the instructions which required nonverbal communication, gesture, and eye contact. The hesitancy continued. The teachers were not used to interacting with each other in this way. After some awkward stumbling, and finally a moment of extreme "failure" in the game, the entire group broke out in laughter. At that moment, the mood of the room shifted. The game continued with increasing enthusiasm and the teachers slowly dropped their resistance and rigidity.*

> *The step of getting on our feet and out of our heads can be a challenge for some groups. Most of us are accustomed to sitting still and using our minds more than our bodies in learning spaces. But accessing our intuitive self, based in our body, along with our rational mind is essential in this work, for it allows participants to progress to deeper work. Within the hour the same teachers who were sitting back in silence were engaging in role-playing activities using both their bodies and voices to take on different characters and practice having real-life conversations with their students.*

> *-Alison Lehner*

3-1

SAFE SPACE TOUR:

IMAGINE SAFER SPACES
THROUGH ACTION AND
REFLECTION.

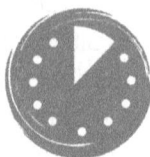

◯ **Bigger Than Us**

▷ **Take Action**

Preparation: Open space to move
Connections: Creative Drama

Steps

1. The facilitator explains that participants will give one another a tour of their school or community. Participants should choose a real place in their lives that they can describe in detail.

2. Have the group divide into pairs, and prompt the participants to decide who will be the first Tour Guide.

3. Ask Tour Guides to lead their tours by physically walking or guiding their partners around the space. Explain that all the tours will happen simultaneously.
   a. Tour Guides share different elements of their space that contribute to it feeling safe—i.e. the bean bag chair they've sat in for years, or the corner of the bed that they read and write on—and take their partner to those places in the room.
   b. Tour Guides should use pantomime to help their partners visualize imaginary new elements of the space.
   c. Ask the Tour Guides to share what they would need to make their space feel even safer.
   d. If there is time, the person taking the tour can ask the Tour Guide questions that invite them to share more details.

4. After 5 to 10 minutes, pause the tours and, as a group, have the participants share the components they imagined that could make their space safer.

5. After the brainstorm, have the participants return to their pairs. The partner who did not lead the last tour now leads a tour of this imagined safe space, using ideas from their brainstorm.

Application

Use this activity to do tours of any place, or help participants envision imaginary worlds.

Reflection Questions

- What were some of the key differences in your first and second space tours?
- What can we do as individuals to make this space safer? What can we do as a community?

Notes

If you haven't already introduced the idea of a safe space, discuss what we mean when we talk about safe spaces, clarifying that this is about more than physical safety.

Encourage participants to layer in all the senses when they give their tours.

If you are worried about crowding and noise, you may opt for fewer tours happening at once. Try dividing into groups of four or five. Or, assign groups to different parts of the space/the building to keep tours spread out, and encourage exploration of different spaces.

3-2

SEATED POWER:

EXAMINE POWER IN RELATIONSHIPS BY USING CHAIRS AND BODY IMAGES.

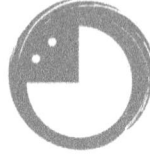

(?) **Does That Count**

(...) **Start The Convo**

Preparation: Open space for performance, one chair, large paper or board to write on
Connections: Theatre of the Oppressed

Steps

1. Ask the group to form an audience, facing a playing space that contains one chair in the center of the room.

2. Invite the group to enter the playing space one at a time and create a **tableau** about Power, using the chair.
   a. In the first round, the participants create a tableau in which they have power over the chair.
   b. In the second round, the participants create a tableau in which the chair has power over them.
   c. In the third round, the participants demonstrate equally shared power with the chair.

3. Choose a particularly dynamic or striking tableau, and invite a second participant into the playing space to take the place of the chair.

4. Now a two-person tableau, invite the audience to write 4 lines of dialogue together out loud. Write their ideas on the butcher paper or chalkboard that tell the story of the image.

5. Choose four lines from the previous brainstorm, and invite the participants in the tableau to improvise a conversation beginning with the lines of dialogue created by the audience.

6. The group may go back and repeat steps 2 through 6, or the facilitator can choose another image from the last round for steps 4 through 5.

Application

At the start of this activity, we deal with abstract images of Power. The chair is not cast as a particular character, nor does it have to be treated literally like a chair.

This activity can be used to interrupt and analyze power dynamics between two characters, or between characters and institutions. For example, in Step 4, the facilitator can cast one participant as a school system that maintains an abstinence-only sex education policy and another participant as a principal who wants to provide comprehensive education to their students.

Reflection Questions

- Was there a moment during this activity that challenged your understanding of Power?
- In the real world, what gives us Power? What takes our Power away?

Notes

It is helpful to warm up for this activity and other tableau work with a low exposure movement game—i.e. Sound and Gesture, activity 1-5 in this book—or some basic physical warm-up.

The images also tend to be more successful when the facilitator insists on poses that are completely "frozen," i.e., no body movements at all.

3-3

THE FIRST TIME I... :

EXPLORE "FIRST" EXPERIENCES THROUGH ANONYMOUS STORYTELLING AND GESTURE.

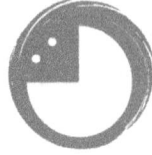

Me We

Start The Convo

Preparation: Writing materials, open space to move

Steps

1. The facilitator introduces the topic of Identity and offers the group a definition.
   a. We use: *"Identities are made up of many overlapping and contradicting feelings—where we come from, who we want to be, what we like, what we don't—and how we act on those feelings."*

2. Ask the participants to write 3 to 5 sentences about a significant "first" moment that informed their identity as it relates to their understanding of sexuality.
   a. This could include: A first kiss, a first moment of sexual desire, or a first time they encountered portrayals of sex in the media.
   b. Remind the participants not to put their names on the story or write anything that would reveal them as the author.

3. Once the participants finish writing, ask them to move about the room, **covering the space**. As they walk, prompt the participants to pass their story to someone new (like passing a note). Without looking at their note, participants then pass it to someone new again, then to someone new again (ensuring anonymity).

4. Make sure that each participant has one story, and instruct the participants to find a spot in the room to read their story silently to themselves.

5. Each participant should take a moment to think of a title for the story they just read. When they have a title in mind, ask them to work independently to create a gesture for that title.

6. Have the group form a circle, and invite the participants to perform the titles and gestures for the full group, one at a time.

7. *Optional extension:* Participants find a partner and share their gestures. Each partner writes down a feeling or phrase that comes to mind when they see the movement. Have the participants share these phrases with the whole group.

8. Ask the group to reflect on the similarities and differences between the stories.

Application

This structure of passing anonymous stories and responding with gesture can be applied to any story prompt.

Reflection Questions

- How did the translation of form (i.e. word to image) impact your understanding of the author's story?
- Which aspects of Identity came up in this activity? Did this activity alter your understanding of identity, particularly as it relates to sex and sexuality?

Notes

The prompt for the stories could be adapted to explore other content areas (shame, power, accountability, etc.).

3-4

SHARE YOUR STRATEGY: CREATE AND EMULATE GESTURES FOR BEING AN ALLY.

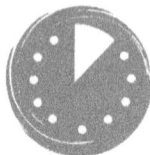

Me We

Take Action

Preparation: Open space to move

Steps
*This activity builds on **1-5: Sound and Gesture.***

1. Gather the participants in a standing circle, and ask everyone to reflect on a moment in which they were an **ally**—a person who sticks up for someone or something they believe in.

2. Each participant creates an abstract sound and gesture that represents that moment.

3. Going around the circle, have the participants share their gestures. After each participant shares, the full group repeats their sound and gesture.

   a. Prompt the participants to observe carefully, and try to memorize at least one sound and gesture aside from their own.

4. Ask one participant to begin by first doing their gesture, and then doing somebody else's, to "send" the gesture to that person.

5. The second person "receives" their gesture by repeating it, and then does the gesture of someone else in the circle.

6. The game play continues with the participants working to pass and receive sounds and gestures as smoothly as possible.

Application

Use this game to explore personal experiences without having to tell long-winded stories. This is a good way to get participants to distill information to its essence. The facilitator could also choose to have the gestures be about a common moment or experience such as, *"A time when you felt safe in your identity,"* or *"something that happened today that made you feel loved."*

Reflection Questions

- What was it like to try on the strategies of others by taking on their sound and gesture?

Notes

Sound and gesture works best when the facilitator insists on no words for the sound portion of the exercise.

For an added challenge, try picking up the pace of the game, or maintaining a steady rhythm as the participants pass and receive.

3-5

I AM A CONDOM:

EXPLORE VARIOUS SETTINGS
WHERE CONVERSATIONS ABOUT
SEXUAL DECISION-MAKING
OCCUR.

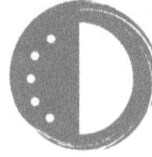

? Does That Count

••• Start The Convo

Preparation: Open space to move
Connections: Improvisational Theatre (based on the game "I Am a Tree," origins unknown)

Steps

1. Have the participants form a standing circle.

2. Ask a participant to step into the middle and freeze in a pose or shape that physically embodies a condom. To establish the pattern of the game, the participant should say, "I am a condom," once they assume the physical pose.

3. Have a second participant enter the circle, and pose as a character or object that could be in a scene with a condom (e.g., "a bed"). The second participant assumes that image and says "I am a [bed]."

4. With 2 images frozen inside the circle, a third person will enter to complete the **tableau** as another character or object that could be in the scene, saying, "I am a ____."

5. Once there is a complete tableau consisting of three characters/objects, instruct the first participant (i.e. "the condom") to choose one person to tap out of the middle. They will then say, "I am a [condom] and I am taking the ____ with me."
    a. The first participant (in this example, the condom), and whoever they tapped out return to the outside of the circle.
    b. There should now be one person left in the middle of the circle. They repeat their phrase, and the group begins to

116

build a new image. Have 2 new participants add themselves to the scene as new objects/characters.

6. Continue the game play and encourage participants to choose new situations that contain different sexual or intimate scenarios.

7. As participants get the hang of the pattern, add "thoughts out loud": Tap a participant on the shoulder and ask for "thoughts out loud" from a person or object in each scene (e.g. "What is this character thinking?" or "What would this object say if it could talk?") to hear how each feels about the situation.

Application

This activity zooms in on relationships and environments and helps us explore conflict in different settings. It can also help us imagine a world or story we would want to see. Through simple frozen images, participants analyze the way that characters and objects might interact or feel about different situations.

Reflection Questions

- Which tableau(s) seemed to present the most challenging scenario when it comes to sexual decision making?
- How might you imagine some of these scenes playing out if we were to add dialogue or movement?

Notes

A sample script for a round of this game is as follows:
1. Person 1: "I am a condom." (enters circle, freezes in image)
2. Person 2: "I am a bed." (enters circle, freezes in image)
3. Person 3: "I am a person waiting in the doorway." (enters circle, freezes in image)
4. Person 1: "I am a condom and I'm taking the bed." (Person 1 and 2 leave the circle)
5. Person 3: "I am a person waiting in the doorway." (the pattern begins again with new images and new volunteers)

For groups who have not had much experience with tableau, it is helpful to warm-up with a low exposure physical activity to get participants comfortable and aware of their bodies.

3-6

RELATIONSHIP STATUES: EXAMINE BODY
LANGUAGE AND POWER
THROUGH STILL IMAGES.

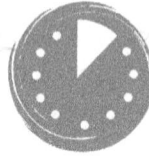

? Does That Count

··· Start The Convo

Preparation: Open space for performance area
Connections: Theatre of the Oppressed

Steps

1. Ask for 2 participants to stand next to each other in the front of the room.

2. Have each participant choose an emotion and an intensity level (high, medium, or low) to freeze in a pose. They should not share this with their partner or the audience.

3. Say "Go" and have the 2 participants strike their poses.

4. While they are frozen, ask the audience what they think the story of this relationship is:

   a. Who are these people? How do they know each other? Who has more power?
   b. How does our physicality affect our interactions with others?

Application

Use this activity to analyze nuances of body language and the ways in which we unintentionally display different levels of power.

Reflection Questions

- How could you tell who had more power in each of these images?
- How does physicality/body language affect our relationships?

Notes

Depending on the group, it may be helpful to establish a scale for high-medium-low before this activity. You could prompt a volunteer to demonstrate an emotion like *joy* at low, medium, and high levels. For a lower exposure option, you could ask the whole group to play through various emotions at various levels simultaneously, either in place, or moving throughout the room.

Sample Facilitation Script

(Note: Before beginning the activity, ask the participants to make a circle, with enough room in the middle for a play space.)

FACILITATOR: *"Let's have two volunteers move into the middle of our circle. Without talking, think of a feeling. Pick one, don't say what it is. Now, choose in your head, how large or intense that feeling is. Are you feeling it just a little? Or a whole lot? Got a feeling and a level in your head?"*

(Have the two volunteers acknowledge they are ready.)

FACILITATOR: *"When I say 'go,' the two of you will make a statue with your body, in other words, strike a pose that embodies the feeling and level of feeling you chose. Ready? Go!"*

(The two volunteers freeze in place.)

FACILITATOR: *Everyone in the circle, let's take a good look at what our players have offered to us. Capture it in your mind! Players, make any adjustments you need to make so you can stay in that position for a few minutes. Audience, who are these people? How do they know each other? Where are they? What are they doing?*

(Allow the audience to either raise hands and answer one at a time, or have free-flowing conversation, depending on their ability to self-manage interruptions.)

FACILITATOR: *Now, looking at their posture and facial expressions: Who has more power? What makes you think so?*

(Take final ideas from the audience. Then allow the players to release their poses, and ask for two new players. Repeat the prompts. After a number of rounds, lead the group in a reflection.)

Sample Reflection and Brainstorming Prompts:

- *What kind of feelings are we identifying as powerful? As weak?*
- *What are we learning about power? What are we missing?*

3-7

MAXIMIZE/ MINIMIZE: Use still

IMAGES TO EXPLORE EMOTIONAL
EXPERIENCES

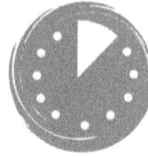

Does That Count

Start The Convo

*Preparation: Prompts (examples in "Application" section), open space
for performance area*
Connections: Improvisational Theatre

Steps

1. Ask the group for an emotion that someone might experience before their first sexual encounter.

2. Invite three participants to come to the front of the room.

3. Ask each participant to make their own statue—a frozen picture with their body—of this emotion.

4. Have the group discuss the differences and similarities between the participants' physicality.

5. Tell the participants that their current statue is a "level 5," the midpoint on a scale from 1 to 10. Ask the participants to MAXIMIZE their pose, increasing its scope and size to a 6, 7, 8, etc.

6. Ask the group when someone might feel the MAXIMUM of this emotion?

7. Repeat the exercise, but have all three participants MINIMIZE, counting them down all the way to a 1.

8. Ask the group when someone might feel the MINIMUM of this emotion?

Application

This game can be modified to explore multiple themes by changing the timeline ticks to things like "Experiences of the media," "Terms you used for anatomical parts," or "Educational milestones."

Reflection Questions

Use this game to embody and explore the emotions that a character, or oneself, might experience while doing any activity, talking to any person, or going to any place. This activity can be adapted for a range of ages; simply adjust the prompts to suit your group's goals and needs.

A few examples:
For middle schoolers:
- What emotion might someone experience while deciding if they are ready to have sex?
- What emotion might someone experience before asking their parent or another adult for a sexuality-related resource?

For high schoolers:
- What emotion might someone experience before going to get tested for STI's?
- What emotion might someone experience before talking to their partner about contraception?
- What emotion might someone experience when interrupting a violent message online/in person?
- In which ways might this emotion help us before our first sexual encounter? In which ways might this emotion be an obstacle?
- How do we move from extreme to moderate feelings? What causes us to move from extreme to moderate emotions? What strategies could we practice, for instance, to calm ourselves down?

Notes

Facilitators can play with changing the variables, such as the number of people who perform or the number of emotions explored (try 2 or 3 at a time!).

3-8

PARTNERED POWER: INVESTIGATE

POWER THROUGH MIRRORING.

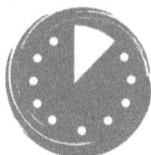

Does That Count

Me We

Preparation: Open space to move
Connections: Theatre of the Oppressed

Steps

1. Ask the participants to stand face-to-face with a partner. Explain that this is a silent activity that requires focus and eye contact.

2. Have the participants choose who is partner A and who is partner B.

3. Prompt partner A to begin moving their body, slowly, in any way at all. Instruct partner B, as best they can, to follow exactly what A is doing, as if they are A's mirror.

4. Allow the game play to continue for at least 2 minutes. Encourage the participants to use body parts other than arms and hands (the easiest). Once the group seems to be comfortable using their whole bodies, prompt partner A to lead the pair, and travel throughout the space.

   a. Encourage partner A to explore height levels (low, medium, high).
   b. Remind the group to keep each other safe by staying aware of other pairs moving through the room.
   c. Remind the group to stay silent while moving throughout the room.

5. Have the participants switch roles so that partner B leads the pair, still moving throughout the space.

6. Ask the pairs to pause. Instruct both partners to lead and follow at once. Tell them that neither should instigate a movement, but decide and move together (still without speaking!).

Application

This activity can explore equitable relationships and lead to a conversation about give and take. It can also apply to a conversation about group think and/or peer pressure.

Reflection Questions

- What was your experience like? Who had power? When? Why?
- How did consent play a role in this game?

Notes

If there is time, and especially with younger people, consider demonstrating with two participants first.

Optional higher stakes extension: Have the partners stand facing each other. Instruct partner B to follow Partner A's hand movements, as if on a string. Have partner A lead Partner B around, in total control, but keeping their partner safe. Then, have the partners switch.

3-9

POWER SHIFT: CREATE
IMAGES AND DIALOGUE THAT
EXPLORE POWER DYNAMICS.

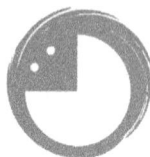

(?) Does That Count

(▶) Take Action

*Preparation: Open space for
performance area*
Connections: Theatre of the Oppressed

Steps
This activity builds on 3-2: Seated Power.

1. Divide the participants into pairs, and ask them to choose one of
   the following ways power might be imbalanced in a relationship.
   Or, ask them to come up with their own.
   a. Level of experience: One partner is a virgin, and the other is
      not
   b. Level of "out-ness": One partner has come out openly as
      gay to their community, and the other partner has not
   c. Money: One partner buys the other gifts and life supplies
   d. Age difference: One partner is much older than the other
   e. Alcohol: One partner is drunker than the other
   f. Gender difference: One partner is a man, and the other is a
      woman, or one partner is cisgender, and the other is
      gender nonconforming.

2. Ask the pairs to use their bodies to create a **tableau** of their
   chosen power imbalance, i.e., the pairs should freeze in a position
   so that, together, they make an image that illustrates the
   imbalance. The image can be literal or metaphorical.

3. Once the pairs have created their tableaus, ask them to generate a
   line of dialogue that would equalize the dynamics of the
   relationship. What could one of these characters say that would
   create a balance of power?

4. Finally, ask the pairs to create a new tableau that better matches
   this line of dialogue.

5. Have the pairs rehearse all three moments: The original tableau, the line of dialogue, and the new tableau.

6. Go around the room and have each pair perform their sequences for the whole group.

Application

Use this activity to examine power imbalances in any relationship (teacher/student, parent/child, doctor/patient, boss/employee, etc.).

This activity can also be useful in bystander intervention contexts, where identifying the problem (as an image) is the first step in interrupting it.

Reflection Questions

- How are power dynamics created?
- What strategies did we use to create equally shared power?
- How realistic did this feel? Why or why not?

Notes

This activity can be stopped at any point after completion of Step 2 if the group is less comfortable with each other. Using the full activity exposes participants at higher levels and also leads to more in-depth conversation about misuse of power.

3-10

3-2-1 ANATOMY!:
ASSESS KNOWLEDGE OF
ANATOMY THROUGH 3-PERSON
IMAGES.

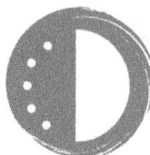

Health 411

Preparation: Anatomy prompts (examples in Step 5)

Steps

1. Split the participants into pairs.

2. Explain that, in just a moment, partners are going to make a silent **tableau** of an object with just their bodies. Both partners must be a part of the frozen picture, creating the same object together (In other words, they should combine their bodies to create the full shape of the object itself, not show a person using the object). Participants will have only 3 seconds to create the statue, as the facilitator counts down from three.

3. Play an example round, having the participants form a tree. Countdown from three: "3-2-1 . . . TREE!"

4. While the pairs stay frozen, invite the participants to glance around at other tableaus with only their eyes. Or, invite half of the participants to unfreeze, and take a quick tour of the tableaus in the room.

5. Continue the game with various anatomy prompts: "Make a statue of a ___. 3-2-1,___!"
    a. Vulva
    b. Penis
    c. Clitoris
    d. Testes
    e. Breasts
    f. Mouth
    g. Ovaries
    h. Fallopian tube

Application

Use this game after a day of content, to test the participants' memory of various anatomical parts. This game is best as a warm-up with a group that's already comfortable with each other.

Reflection Questions

- Why do you think conversations about anatomy, like this game, can get silly or uncomfortable?
- In your opinion, why is learning about anatomy an important part of sexual health/sexuality education?

Notes

There may be a lot of giggles during this game, but that's part of the fun! Keep the pace moving by keeping to the strict 3-second time frame, and challenging students to freeze in their tableau, if only for a few seconds.

If 3 seconds seems tricky for some of the more complicated prompts, try extending the time to 5 or 10 seconds.

3-11

MOVING IDENTITIES: EMBODY AND EXPLORE VARIOUS IDENTITIES AND THE WAYS THEY INTERSECT.

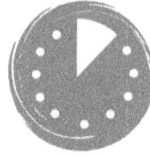

Me We

Start The Convo

Preparation: Open space to move
Connections: Improvisational Theatre (see "Lone Wolf" by Viola Spolin)

Steps

1. Have the participants brainstorm a list of different kinds of identities they assume in their own lives (male, cis woman, daughter, genderqueer, etc.).

2. Ask the participants to spread out in the room. Have each participant strike a frozen pose of one of their identities. Encourage them to exaggerate their poses.

3. Tap one participant to begin moving around the room, embodying their exaggerated identity. This person can make any kind of movements, but must eventually freeze and "give" their moving energy to one of the other frozen statues.

   a. For the energy hand-off to work, all participants must be fully present, and the participant who is moving should pass their energy with intention, making sure to use eye contact.

4. Prompt the statue who receives the energy to then unfreeze, and move around the room in their identity, until they, too, give the energy to another frozen statue.

5. For more advanced groups, participants can also play with "take," where a frozen statue begins to move, and forces the currently-moving statue to freeze. In both versions, remind the group that only one participant should be moving at all times.

Application

This activity is a way to allow participants to isolate and try on different labels they might use, and see what kind of energy those identities bring to a space.

Reflection Questions

- How did our different identities interact? Did they influence one another?
- How did it feel to exaggerate an aspect of your (or someone else's) identity?
- How did it feel to see aspects of your (or someone else's) identity exaggerated?
- Did you observe any stereotypes in this game? How did you navigate the tendency to fall into a stereotype?

Notes

To avoid stereotyping identities, make sure to have participants to play first with only identities they carry themselves.

If the group is ready, the facilitator may move into having participants represent identities they do not personally carry. Be sure to frame this exercise, and follow up with a conversation on representation and stereotype.

For groups/facilitators new to on-your-feet physical activities like this one, the energy hand-off may require a bit of practice. This aspect of the game is a challenge that should help hone group listening and presence, and ultimately strengthen the sense of ensemble.

3-12

CAN WE TOUCH YOU: PRACTICE ASKING FOR AND RESPONDING TO PHYSICAL CONSENT.

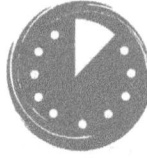

Me We

Does That Count

Preparation: Open space to move
Connections: Devised Theatre (adapted from "Walk, Stop, Drop," from Michael Rohd)

Steps

1. Invite the participants to move around the room, and **cover the space** by simple walking.

2. After 30 to 60 seconds, the facilitator says, "When one person in the room stops, we will all stop." Practice this as a group. Then say, "When one person in the room starts moving again, we all move." Play with stop and start for 30 to 60 seconds.

3. Then, add the next layer: "When one person drops, we all drop." Demonstrate this by crouching to the ground or bending down and instructing others to crouch as well. Then say, "When one person picks it up and starts walking again, we all walk." Play with stop and drop for a minute or so.

4. The facilitator pauses the room by stopping, just as they would in the game. The facilitator then says, "At any point in time, someone can stop and point to someone else in the room. When one person points, we all point. That person will then ask, 'Can we touch you?' If the person getting pointed to says, 'Yes,' we will all move towards the pointee, and touch them on their shoulder at the same time. If they say 'No,' we simply continue moving through space."

5. Continue playing with stop, drop, and "Can we touch you?"

Application

This activity is a way to allow participants to experience what it feels like to ask for, give, receive, and deny consent in a non-sexual context.

Reflection Questions

- How did it feel when someone said no? When they said yes?
- How did it feel to have someone ask if they could touch you?
- Did anybody feel pressure to respond in a particular way?
- What does this have to do with consent as it applies to sex?

Notes

This is a game that can be taught in stages and/or repeated at multiple points for added reinforcement. It is important as a facilitator to keep things active and moving. Insisting that everybody touch the person at the *exact same moment* adds another level of challenge for the group.

The goal is to practice consent in a fun, safe way. If a group seems uncomfortable with the activity, the facilitator can build up to it with lower-exposure activities around consent.

CHAPTER 4 - ACT IT OUT

You've built a supportive community. Your participants have shared diverse stories and perspectives. Your group is comfortable moving and exploring its potential. Now it's time to put these ideas into action. After all, there's quite a gap between knowing what you *intend* to do and actually *doing* it.

Often, what stands in our way is a fear of failure. A young person who feels insecure might be scared of asking their crush on a date. A boy who doesn't want to seem inexperienced, or uncool, might not know how to suggest using a condom. A girl who feels shame about her sexual history or confused about her options might feel silenced in a doctor's office.

In a supportive setting, the community you have built can help the possibility of failure feel safe—or at least okay. This sense of possible failure, in fact, is key: Young people need a safe space to practice acting out *what might be*, and they need permission to get it wrong a few times. Acting out imaginary scenarios helps young people gain realistic language and practical tools that will be useful in real life. As a group, we can try on language and possibilities for conflict resolution, because the ethos is ripe for "failure" to be safe.

> We were sitting on folding chairs in a church basement—four performers (including myself), a small group of adult mentors, and about 50 young people from across the city. We were gathered together for a short, performance-based sexual health workshop hosted by a local youth enrichment program. Many of the students came from religious families, and immediately we were met with resistance for the idea that they were even going to talk about sex as middle schoolers. "That's nasty!" "Why do we have to talk about this?"
>
> But as students were introduced to the characters in the play, they became so engrossed in the scenes and deeply committed to watching the characters succeed, that all their reluctance fell away. As I crouched in a small group of students, brainstorming ways that my character could more easily talk to his girlfriend about sex, one of the students called out "Just take her to Jamba Juice!"—as if this were the most normal and necessary idea in the world. We all laughed, imagining two awkward

young lovers discussing their protective options while sipping on strawberry-banana smoothies. The air had lightened.

Through the ability to play perspective within this scenario, the students came to appreciate a new perspective and try on a possible solution without fear of real-life consequences, judgment, or failure.
- Jacob Watson

4-1

CONNECT AND PROTECT: INTERVIEW STI PROTECTION METHODS TO CHOOSE THE RIGHT ONE FOR DIFFERENT PEOPLE AND CONTEXTS.

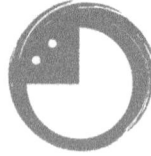

Health 411

Preparation: Fact sheets and character scenario slips for all participants, open space to move
Connection: Creative Drama

Steps

1. Frame this activity by explaining that even if we know all the facts about the types of protection that exist, it can still be hard to choose which method is best for us. This **game** helps us become experts in choosing.

2. Split the group in Group A and Group B. Give members of Group A a fact sheet on one of the following methods of STI protection:
   a. **Abstinence**
   b. Monogamy
   c. Internal/Female condoms
   d. External/Male condoms
   e. Dental dams

3. Have each member from Group B pull 2 different qualities from the scenario grab bag. The scenario grab bag should include the following factors, printed on one per slip.
   a. Latex allergy
   b. Can't spend any money on STI protection
   c. Comfortable talking to a doctor about STI protection
   d. Comfortable talking to a trusted adult about STI protection
   e. Uncomfortable talking to ANY adults about STI protection
   f. One partner already has an STI
   g. Willing to try sexual activities that don't include penetration

     h.   Want to prevent pregnancy
     i.   Comfortable talking to their partner about STI protection
     j.   Uncomfortable talking to their partner about STI protection

4. Give Group B a minute to look at their papers. Explain that, working independently, Group A will choose 2 pros and 2 cons for their method that they can share quickly (they should write them down if they need help remembering).

5. Meanwhile, Group B, working independently, will imagine that they are a person who has the 2 qualities listed on the paper slips in their hands. Each member of Group B will write down 2 questions their character could ask to find the best method of STI protection for them.
    a. After a minute, instruct the groups to get up and walk around the room. Tell Group B members to look for people from Group A and ask them their questions to see if it's a good fit. Tell Group A members to look for folks from Group B who they can convince to use their method of STI protection.
    b. The goal is for everyone to find a good match; in other words, which method of protection (Group A) is most compatible with the character's circumstances and questions (Group B).

Application

This activity helps participants think through real-life applications of protection methods.

Reflection Questions

- Why is your pair a good match?
- What were some potential bad matches you encountered?

Notes

This activity can be used with no prior STI information but works best if participants already have some ability to identify risk-reduction methods.

THE SEX ED PLAYBOOK

4-2

MYTH BUSTING:
RESPOND TO STI-RELATED MYTHS THROUGH DIALOGUE AND ROLE-PLAY.

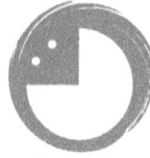

Health 411

Preparation: STI myth handouts (1 for each pair/group), seated writing areas, open space for performance area

Steps

1. Have each member from Group B pull 2 different qualities from the scenario grab bag. The scenario grab bag should include the following factors, printed on one per slip.
   a. It's my first time, so I can't get an STI.
   b. We only have oral sex, so I don't need to worry about STIs.
   c. You can get HIV from kissing.
   d. My partner looks all right, so we don't have anything to worry about.
   e. If I get an STI, no one will want to have sex with me ever again.
   f. It's okay not to tell my partner I have an STI as long as I'm not showing any symptoms while we're hooking up.

2. Prompt the participants to imagine that someone said this message to them. Ask them to write down 4 lines of conversation that they would say in response that correct or support the message.

3. Have the pairs to perform their conversations for the class.

Application

This activity allows participants to put learned STI content into their own words and model interruptions of incorrect information.

Reflection Questions

- What strategies seemed to work best to interrupt the myths?
- Why do you think myths about STIs (and sex in general) come about in the first place?

Notes

This activity can also work in small groups instead of pairs.

Depending on the group, the facilitator may want to go through an example scene first to establish some "best practices" together for myth busting in a way that is sex-positive and shame reducing.

4-3

TRANSFORMING OPPRESSIVE MESSAGES: PLAY OUT VARIOUS INTERRUPTION STRATEGIES TO STOP OPPRESSIVE LANGUAGE AND BEHAVIOR.

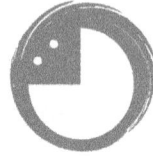

Start The Convo

Take Action

Preparation: Writing materials, open space to move
Connections: Theatre of the Oppressed

Steps

1. Instruct participants to write on slips of paper one or more oppressive messages (homophobic, racist, sexist, transphobic, classist, ableist, etc.) that they struggled to interrupt or challenge. Encourage the group to write in the voice of the person who spoke the message. So not: "I heard Jack say Jill was asking for it because of her skirt length." But rather: "Did you see what Jill was wearing? She's asking for it."

2. Gather ideas from the group to generate a list of interruption tactics. Explain that at this moment we are not looking for direct responses or quotes, but *ways* of responding: Like 'Ask a Question' or 'Use We-Centered Language.' *(Refer to the "Interruption Tactics" listed in the introduction.)*

3. Have the participants form a standing circle. Ask for two volunteers to play out the first interruption in the middle of the circle.

4. Assign one volunteer as "A" to represent the perspective of the oppressive message, while assigning the second volunteer as "B" to attempt to interrupt that message, and transform A's perspective. When the facilitator says, "Go," both volunteers will play out the scene. Let the other participants know that anyone in

the circle can tag out either A or B during the conversation and continue the dialogue using their own tactics.

5. Invite person A to begin the role-play by sharing their negative or oppressive message. B can use any of the tactics the group brainstormed to respond. Encourage participants on the outside of the circle to tap in with new ideas to complicate the scene throughout.

6. When the group is out of ideas or the scenario seems resolved, clap to clear the circle. Invite two new people to step into the center and begin a new dialogue with a new message.

Application

The messages used can be curated depending on group needs. Perhaps the group encounters racist language while door-knocking during a political campaign; the facilitator can mine messages directly from that experience. Or perhaps the group is working to address homophobia in their school; the group can directly pull messages heard from their peers.

Reflection Questions

- Which modes of interruption did you think were most effective? Why?
- What was it like to play through scenes as practice for real life? How do you think you'll apply this exercise in your own life?

Notes

Depending on the group, the facilitator may opt to enter into Step 2 with a pre-populated list of strategies, rather than starting from scratch. Share a list of 3 to 5 ideas that model strong tactics, and invite the participants to discuss, tweak, and add to this list.

Note that the goal of interrupting oppressive language is to change hearts and minds, not to shut people down. Emphasize that in order to invite others into our beliefs and values, we want to transform oppressive language rather than simply shut it up. Explain that as we practice using these, we'll observe which tactics facilitate transformation and which ones facilitate deeper conflict. Allowing participants to swap in and out keeps the volunteers safe and helps the group recognize a broad range of approaches to resolving the conflict.

It is important to encourage students not to make fun of the perspective of the oppressor when playing it out. Making a caricature of that person will lead to continual stereotyping and prevent players from exploring the strongest interruption tactics. Suggest that we treat this as an exercise in compassion. The person speaking the oppressive message should not judge the message as they deliver it, but rather exercise curiosity about why someone might believe that idea. Feel free to reflect on each dialogue before moving on to another.

4-4

CHANCE CONFLICTS: ROLE-PLAY
THROUGH DIFFICULT
CONVERSATIONS USING
GROUP-GENERATED QUOTES.

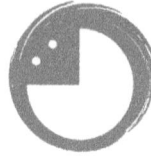

Me We

Take Action

Preparation: Slips of paper (1 for each student), open space for performance area

Steps

1. Guide the group in choosing the "where/what/who" of a difficult sexuality conversation, including a setting, conflict, and characters. The characters should be a young person (player A) and one of their "influences" (player B). Influences may be any person or place that affects how we think or act when it comes to sex (e.g. parents, teacher, the media).

2. Assign half the group to write as Player A and half to write as Player B. On their own slips of paper, have the participants write a quote from the perspective of their assigned character. For Player A, write a question the young person might ask. For Player B, write something the influence might say that could be an "obstacle" for the young person.

3. Collect the slips, keeping Player A and Player B quotes in separate piles.

4. Invite two volunteers to the playing space to play through the scene, one as Player A and the other as Player B. Give each volunteer a slip of paper appropriate for the character they will play, face side down. Instruct participants not to look at their slips yet.

5. Explain that Player A and Player B will begin improvising a conversation, using the setting, conflict, and characters agreed upon earlier by the group. After the improvisation has gone on a

moment, the facilitator taps one partner on the shoulder. When a player feels the tap, they will speak the sentence on their slip.

6. With everyone aware of the rules of play, Player A and Player B can begin playing through their scene.

    a. The players are not allowed to sort through and choose the slip they like, but instead must read the slip at the top of their pile. This is part of the challenge!
    b. Their scene partner must react, and both must continue the conversation with the new question or obstacle that is now part of the dialogue.

7. As the game play ensues, the facilitator may continue to tap the same pair, adding different obstacles and dimensions to their scene. Or, the facilitator may rotate through with new volunteers at any point.

Application

This activity can be applied to any kind of difficult conversation between any two people. The more specific the group is about setting, character, and conflict, the stronger the scene will be.

Reflection Questions

- Remember that Player A should stay focused on their goal or purpose in the imagined scenario and not "give up" when faced with obstacles. In other words, what is driving their character in the scene(s) we just saw and played through? Did they achieve their goal? Why or why not?
- Were there any moments from this activity you'd want to use in approaching difficult conversations in your life?

Notes

After participants write "obstacles," unpack the word. Could an obstacle be a judgment? A punishment? A difficult question? A strong difference of opinion?

4-5

SEXUAL SCRIPTS:

BREAK DOWN POPULAR SCRIPTS
BY SPEAKING IN CLICHÉ.

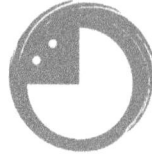

? **Does That Count**

▶ **Take Action**

*Preparation: Large paper or board
to write on, open space to move and for performance area*

Steps

1. Lead a group brainstorm by first creating a chart with three
   columns labeled "Foreplay/Before" "The Act/During" and "The
   Aftermath." Discuss sexual scripts with the group. What are the
   scripts we receive from the media for how to be sexual? In the
   most clichéd romantic comedy you can think of, what do we see in
   the Foreplay scene? What always happens? What about The Act?
   And the Aftermath?

   a. Gather suggestions for ingredients in the foreplay scene.
      (e.g. candles, roses, alcohol, etc.).
   b. Gather suggestions for ingredients in the actual sex scene
      (e.g. clothes ripping off, dramatic female orgasm, no
      condoms, etc.).
   c. Gather suggestions for ingredients in the scene after the
      sex scene (e.g. regret, one person sneaking out, breakfast
      in bed, etc.).

2. Explain to the group that they will create one-minute, two-person
   scenes that name what lies beneath the surface of romantic
   comedies. Each scene should include at least one cliché from each
   of the three parts of the group brainstorm. Instruct the
   participants to use suggestions from the brainstorm as the
   primary dialogue, as opposed to realistic dialogue they might see
   in a real movie scene. For example, 'Lighting candles' might be the
   first line of a text between two characters, followed by the line, "A
   dozen roses!" Also explain that when they create these scenes, the
   dialogue should be paired with big, bold gestures (again, not
   realistic staging like they would see in a movie).

3. Divide the group up into pairs. Prompt the participants to find some open space in the room to work with their partner to craft their scene.

4. Bring the group back together to have the pairs each share their scene. Discuss each of the scenes with the group.

Application

This activity can be used to highlight the scripts and habits of any cultural institution. Asking participants to write dialogue that only uses the language of cliché and dominant narrative helps viewers understand the ways in which that language limits us. This activity can apply to thinking beyond the dominant narratives of the reproductive justice movement, or to thinking about common experiences of sexuality education, or to any popular scripted story with a beginning, middle, and end.

Reflection Questions

- What do these scenes teach us about sexual scripts and the media?
- What do they teach us about sexual violence?

Notes

This activity is not about simulating actual sex acts! In order to highlight clichés and underlying problematic scripts we see in movies and other media, it is important that these scenes not seem realistic or "sexy." Both the fun and the power in this activity comes through the style noted in the description. You may even think of the finished scenes as pieces of clown work or commedia dell'arte.

It is possible to create these scenes without including any physical contact between scene partners, so you may add this as a modification if you are worried about the group's comfort level. Another modification is to stage one scene all together with two volunteer performers. In this version, you can take suggestions from the audience, while situating them as the scene's directors.

Finally, we advise that you give pairs enough time to feel confident with what they've made but not so much time that they start to get bored or second-guess their ideas (depending on your group, this might be anywhere from 3-10 minutes).

4-6

MAKE A CHOICE:
MODEL EFFECTIVE
DECISION-MAKING BY PLAYING
OUT MULTIPLE APPROACHES TO
A SCENARIO.

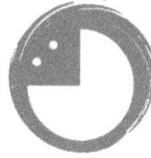

Start The Convo

Take Action

Preparation: Large paper or board to write on, open space to move and for performance area

Steps

1. Ask the participants to name scenarios in which a character has to make a decision about how to behave sexually (i.e. decision to engage in any sexual behavior including kissing or **abstinence**, decision to use protection, decision to tell a friend or parent, etc.). Gather a few suggestions from the group, then select one scenario to explore in depth.

2. With the group, brainstorm 3 different options for how the chosen scenario could play out, depending on choices the character could make. (For example: Tell your partner you are ready to have sex, talk to your partner about waiting to have sex, or avoid the subject.) Make sure to clarify when and where each of these scenarios takes place.

3. Ask for two volunteers to play through different outcomes for this scenario. Prompt the two volunteers to identify which option they are going to play out first, without telling the group, and set up the playing space as necessary. The pair performs their scenario.

4. Have the group reflect on what they just saw. The facilitator may have the same pair play through the remaining two scenarios, or rotate through two more pairs.

5. Once the group has played through all the scenarios, lead a discussion about the positive and negative outcomes for each scenario. Ask the group which choice they would make realistically.

Is it the same or different from the choice they would make ideally?

Application

This activity is useful when exploring any decision-making process and to play through options free from fear of failure.

Reflection Questions

- Why do you think decision-making can be so challenging when it comes to sex? When is it the most difficult? When is it easiest?
- What does improvisation have to do with decision-making in real life? Aside from this exercise, what are other strategies that may help support us in real life decision-making?

Notes

As with other improv-based activities, this one might call for some warm-ups and refreshers on how we can set ourselves and our partners up for success in improv.

4-7

OBSTACLES IN THE ROAD: PRACTICE

OVERCOMING CHALLENGES TO SEXUAL HEALTH.

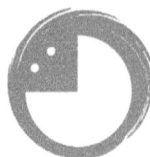

Bigger Than Us

Take Action

Preparation: Large paper or board to write on, open space for "alley" style audience configuration (audience seated on either side of a long, narrow playing space)

Steps

1. Ask for one participant to be a character in a role-play about a young person's journey to get an STI test at the neighborhood clinic.
   a. Optional: Ask, *What is the character's name? What do we know about this person?*

2. Lead a group brainstorm: *What obstacles might this person encounter? Who might oppose them?* Generate and record at least 3 ideas (e.g. the character's mom, who finds out that the character wants an STI test, and gets angry; or the secretary at the clinic's front desk who asks for insurance, but the person doesn't have any.)

3. Choose another participant to play opposite the first player, presenting the first obstacle (e.g. the angry mom).

4. As the participants play out the scene, encourage the main character to try, in as many ways as possible, to overcome the obstacle presented by the second player.

5. When the scene comes to a resolution (or once it has gone on long enough to no longer hold interest), choose *another* participant to be a new scene partner for the main character, presenting a new obstacle from the brainstorm.

6. Have the participants continue to introduce obstacles until the character achieves their goal, or the group feels their story has come to a satisfying stopping point.

Application

Try this activity with different goals for the protagonist. Think about real spaces they might want to go to (e.g. a doctor's appointment, a pro-choice rally, a boyfriend/girlfriend's house), or tasks they may want to achieve (e.g. buy condoms, start a school campaign against **sexual violence**, stick up for an LGBTQ friend).

Reflection Questions

- What were some strong moments on the part of the protagonist that you might want to try when encountering obstacles in real life?

Notes

Try this activity in an "alley" configuration with audience/class seats on either side of the room and a long playing space in the middle. This is useful to map the main character's journey through time and space. Place the first scene and obstacle in the far back of the space, the next scene slightly closer to the middle of the space, the next scene closer to the front … charting the protagonist's forward-moving journey.

As with other improv-based activities, this one might call for some warm-ups and refreshers on how we can set ourselves and our partners up for success in improv.

4-8

HACK THE CIRCLE:

PRACTICE OVERCOMING CHALLENGES TO SEXUAL HEALTH.

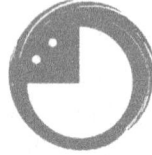

◎ **Bigger Than Us**

▶ **Take Action**

Preparation: A complex scenario that includes at least two characters and a setting.
Connections: Creative Drama

Steps
*This activity builds on **4-3: Transforming Oppressive Messages.***

1. Have the participants form a standing circle.

2. Introduce and review the characters and setting for the scenario the group will explore. It's best if the topic is complex, multifaceted, and sustains multiple points of view. The scenario could be chosen in advance by the facilitator or emerge naturally from conversations or brainstorming with the group. Some examples could be:
   a. A teacher and a pregnant student in conflict over how best to continue her participation in class.
   b. A young person trying to tell their parent about a same-sex partner.
   c. A student approaching another student about something inappropriate or offensive that they heard in the hallway.

3. Ask for two participants to volunteer to play out the scene in the middle of the circle. Let the participants on the outside know that they are "on deck" but should be silent for now. Instruct the volunteers to begin the scene.

4. Once the scene has played out once, ask the volunteers to rewind and play it again. Place a chair in the circle and explain that this time, anybody on the outside can enter the space, and sit in this "thoughts out loud" chair. When that happens, the actors in the middle will pause and listen to the person in the chair, who will

speak the internal thoughts of one of the two characters. The scene will then resume when the person in the chair returns to the circle, with the volunteers incorporating the new information they received from the "thoughts out loud" chair.

   a. Encourage participants to speak in the first person while in the chair — so, to say, "I feel scared" rather than, "I think she is feeling scared."

5. At any point during round two, or in an additional replaying of the scene, the facilitator can introduce the next feature: The interruption circle. Here, anybody on the outside can tap one of the volunteers on the inside and take their role. The new volunteer should continue the scene as the same character with the same perspective, but offer new ideas and solutions to the scenario.

6. Finally, the group can explore how this scenario might play out and impact other people in these characters' lives. To do this, the facilitator can lead a round of bystander thoughts-out-loud, in which the facilitator goes person-by-person around the circle asking for one line of internal thought from somebody who might be witnessing or hearing about the conversation later. For instance, what might the student's mother, or the teacher's co-worker, think of what is happening? Again, encourage these responses in the first person.

7. If the group is advanced, the facilitator could try placing one of these characters into the circle itself, in a new scene with one of the existing characters. This can be repeated as long as it feels useful. Make sure to keep the participants in the scenes limited to 2 people, or things can quickly get unwieldy.

Application

This activity allows you and your participants to dig deep into complex situations, and appreciate them from multiple perspectives. By allowing different people to voice the characters, we can explore all of the different reasons why they might be doing what they are doing.

This activity is especially good at building empathy for viewpoints that we might not like very much or understand, and brainstorming ways to move toward resolution.

You can lead participants through all of these steps, or just some of them. You can also mix and match, and use them at different points in your curriculum. Choose what makes the most sense for the particular conversation and moment at hand.

Reflection Questions

- What were some moments that surprised you during this activity?
- Why do you think [name of character] did [action from the scene]?
- Which characters was it easier to empathize with? Which ones made it harder?
- Could we apply anything that was said during this activity in our own lives?

Notes

One tendency to watch out for right away is the impulse to villainize the "bad guy" in the scenario. Make sure to explain that, although it is hard, we need to try to portray all characters as honestly as possible. Encourage participants to be reflective about why somebody might have a certain perspective, or ask for suggestions about what that character might actually do/say in this scenario.

As you coach the improvisational scenes, encourage them to find a balance of conflict and resolution. Without conflict, the situation will deflate and seem too easy. Without resolution, things will fester and seem impossible. Make sure participants include a bit of both. (One way to do this is to pause the situation and introduce either new obstacles or reasons for one character to ease up.)

As with other improv-based activities, this one might call for some warm-ups and refreshers on how we can set ourselves and our partners up for success in improv.

A FINAL WORD

In our collective teaching artistry and health education work together, we have seen the powerful effect that participatory theatre has on increasing brave and bold engagement in sexuality education contexts. The experienced **pleasure** of participatory theatre uniquely kept the youth we worked with in difficult conversations for long periods of time, made them feel comfortable to ask questions and explore possibilities, and cultivated humor to debunk awkwardness. Opportunities to explore diverse **perspectives** led to a shame-free space where these youth felt their own identities amplified, while empathizing with identities that they did not share. When youth were able to perceive that the ideas they explored in role-play were not their own but their character's ideas, they asked questions without fear of judgment. In **practicing** for real life without fear of failure, youth acted as their most courageous and critical selves. They were able to ask the questions they needed to ask, and explore the scenarios they needed to explore. In sharing **power** with youth through participatory theatre exchanges, we watched them speak up more regularly, indicating that shared power helps youth recognize the value of their own voice.

As a reader of this book, you are joining in a wave of reinventing the way we educate our young people about sexual health. The sooner that we realize the importance of cultural practice and participatory theatre in sexuality education, the sooner we set students up for success in their relationships and lives. It is time to retire the tired and ineffective strategies of the past. Thank you for helping to form a new thread and a new way, and for providing our youth a positive experience in sexuality education, one which will enhance their future and the health of our communities.

APPENDICES

A. Sample Activity Playlists

In the Introduction, we provided some pointers for crafting your curriculum (using activity categories, level of exposure, and content tags). What follows are some sample activity playlists that we invite you to try as you adapt this curriculum to your own needs and objectives. These were created with 45 minute to one hour long sessions in mind and should leave time for discussion and reflection between and after each activity.

The First Day of a Residency
The first day is important because it sets the tone for all the sessions that follow. We recommend preceding these activities by learning participants' names and establishing group agreements at the start of a new residency.
- Four Corners
- Can We Touch You?
- Memory Timeline

Building Ensemble and Trust
While ensemble and trust-building are at the heart of all our activities, you may wish to address these objectives early in the residency, or step back and devote time to them when it seems wanted or needed in your group.
- Safe Space Tour
- Sociogram
- Affinity Group Story Weaving
- Chance Conflicts

Making Change: Identifying and Addressing Issues in Your Community
With the right time, care, and support, the activities in this Playbook can make an impact beyond the walls of your classroom or community space. Use these activities and others in this book to tackle pressing issues in your local community.
- Power Shift
- Social Media Interruptions or Transforming Oppressive Messages
- Break Up Letters to Sexual Violence

Generating Stories and Shareable Material

There are innumerable ways to generate narrative material. In this particular playlist, the second and third activity allow discussion and practice of two key elements of storytelling: relationship and conflict.

- I am a Condom or The First Time I ...
- Relationship Statues
- The Obstacle Road
- Story Fire

Exploring Contraception

You may want to group activities around content areas. Consider this playlist to complement comprehensive instruction about the different forms of contraception, and the pros and cons of each. You may opt for "Sexy Word Association" as something quick and upbeat to help get relevant vocabulary out in the room, and perhaps challenge the group to use words related to contraception or pregnancy.

- Sexy Word Association
- Contraception Speaks
- Make a Choice

Unpacking Sexual Violence

This playlist can help groups begin to explore the concepts of consent and power in a curriculum focusing on sexual violence or healthy relationships. "Sexual Scripts" can open up a conversation about where we receive violent messages, and how we might change them. You might consider other culminating exercises depending on what kind of conversation or creative material you hope to generate. The physical work in Power Shift/Seated Power, for instance, might lead to interesting scenarios that might warrant extra exploration, with an activity like Hack the Circle.

- Yes
- Seated Power
- Power Shift
- Sexual Scripts

B. Glossary

Abstinence
A method of STI or Pregnancy prevention that involves *abstaining* or avoiding activities that have a higher risk of transmitting STIs or fertilizing an egg. Abstinence can mean different things to different people, from avoiding any sexual contact whatsoever, to choosing anal over vaginal penetrative sex. For this reason, it's necessary for partners to communicate clearly around expectations for abstinence to have any efficacy.

Affinity Groups
Groups that share like traits based on identity, dress, or other descriptors, i.e. people with brown hair, people wearing sneakers, indigenous people, elders.

Ally
A person who sticks up for someone or something they believe in.

Boundaries
Refers to delineations between what we desire and what we do not. We may have boundaries around things we find uninteresting, uncomfortable, painful, or triggering. Boundaries can apply to physical as well as emotional or intellectual ways of relating to another person.

Bystander intervention
Any action someone might take to prevent harm from happening to someone else. Harm in this case might be emotional or physical.

Consent
Verbal, enthusiastic, active agreement between two or more parties to ensure mutually beneficial (and pleasurable!) sexual activity.

Contraception
The use of a barrier or hormonal method to prevent pregnancy or STI transmission.

Cover the space
This refers to when a group walks or moves around the space with no particular structure during an activity. If we imagine the room is a plate

balanced on a pole, participants' movements should keep the plate balanced (rather than all clumping on one side).

Game
A structure within which shared goals, elevated stakes, and play can coexist. Games + Story = Participatory theatre.

Gender
The societal and cultural expectations for how people should look and behave. Gender identity is how we, in our heads, think about ourselves. This may match the gender we were assigned at birth, and it may not. It also may match our assigned sex (anatomy and chromosomes), and it may not.

Gender Expression
How a person chooses to share their gender identity. Common means of gender expression include hairstyle, clothing choices, speech patterns, extracurricular activities, and more. There is no wrong way to express any gender, indeed there are infinite ways to do so.

Gender Identity
How a person feels on the inside about their gender. This may or may not align with the assigned sex by a doctor at birth (i.e. their anatomy and chromosomes).

"Get in flow"
This term was coined by Hungarian psychologist Mihaly Csikszentmihalyi, and refers to a highly focused mental state. Group and individual play can bring about this state, which we might also call getting "in the groove" or "in the zone."

Healthy Sexuality, core tenets
We aim to define healthy sexual behavior as objectively as possible, by looking to these three anchors: **safety, consent,** and **pleasure.**
- Safe: *Is the behavior informed by sound, comprehensive medical information? Does it risk causing significant physical or emotional harm?*
- Consensual: *Is there active, enthusiastic consent from all parties involved?*
- Pleasurable: *Is it enjoyable? (Enough said!)*

Levels of Exposure
Levels of exposure is a term to refer to the amount of vulnerability and intensity that participants might experience when engaging in an activity. See the levels defined in more detail in the introduction of this book.

Microaggression
The everyday slights and insults that make a person feel excluded or unwelcome based on various identities they may hold (race, age, gender, sexual orientation, etc.). Microaggressions are often unintentional and symptomatic of cultural beliefs that allow oppression to continue.

The 4 Ps of Participatory Theatre
The four elements of Participatory Theatre are **pleasure**, **perspective**, **power,** and **practice**. Together they create an engaging and democratic learning environment.

Participatory Theatre
An interactive, dialogical mode of performance, in which facilitators and participants co-construct and manipulate narratives through inquiry and play.

Popcorn-style
A method of sharing ideas spontaneously in a group. Without calling on individual participants, whoever feels moved to share does so, one after another, like kernels of corn popping up when they are just hot enough.

Popular education
A mode of learning popularized by Paulo Friere in which teachers and students share power equally, and students drive the priorities and content of lessons.

Reproductive Justice
Reproductive Justice is a sex positive approach that links sexuality, health, and human rights to social justice movements by placing abortion and reproductive health issues in the larger context of the well-being and health of individuals, families, and communities. The mother of Reproductive Justice, SisterSong, defines it as the human right to maintain personal bodily autonomy, to have children, to not have children, and to parent the children we have in safe and sustainable communities.

Resilience
The capacity to recover from obstacles, trauma, or hardship.

Safe space
An environment where all participants trust they will not be intentionally harmed or triggered by other participants and that there will be time and space to talk through harm if it occurs.

Sex (Assigned)
What we are assigned at birth by doctors or parents, based on chromosomal and/or anatomical make up (i.e. XX = female, XY = male.)

Sex-positive
An approach (to education, to life!) that acknowledges the potential positives and power inherent in healthy sexuality, as well as the many diverse forms healthy sexuality can take.

Sexual Health
The state of physical, emotional, and social well-being in relation to sexuality. Sexual health requires a positive and respectful approach to **sexuality** and sexual relationships, as well as the possibility of having pleasurable and safe sexual experiences, free of coercion, discrimination, and violence.

Sexual Orientation
Who we are attracted to; who we want to share our hearts and bodies with.

Sexual Violence
Anything that uses power or control to hurt our bodies or sexual health.

Sexuality
Includes a person's sexual orientation, identity, and relationship to desire and sexual behavior. Sexuality is shaped by physical, chemical, emotional/intellectual, social/interpersonal, and cultural factors, and impacts the way we experience and move through the world.

Shame
An intense negative emotion resulting from a person experiencing failure in relation to their own or other people's standards, feeling responsible for that failure, and believing that failure reflects an inadequate self.

Soft focus
Soft focus is when we allow our eyes to soften and relax so that instead of focusing on one or two things, we can now take in many things at once. This allows us to take the pressure off of our eyes and to gather more information in a new way, including multiple senses.

Stakes
Here, stakes is used to mean the level of investment or risk inherent in an activity.

Stigma
An undesirable attribute in a person that sets that person apart from society.

Tableau
When participants freeze in poses to create an image.

Virginity
An imagined state of value assigned to not having participated in a sexual activity. The given sexual activity may vary from person to person (i.e. penetrative vaginal intercourse, oral sex, penetrative anal intercourse, first pleasurable sexual encounter, first encounter that expresses a person's sexual orientation, etc.).

Yes, and
A mindset and approach made popular by improvisational theatre, in which the group agrees to affirm and add on to each other's ideas, rather than rejecting them or critiquing them right away. (While *yes, and* doesn't mean we have to agree all the time or allow harmful things to be said, it does mean acknowledging what has been said and working to engage with it as generously as possible.)

C. Endnotes

Why Participatory Theatre: A Case for Creative Sexuality Education

1. Glik, Deborah, Glen Nowak, Thomas Valente, Karena Sapsis, and Chad Martin. "Youth Performing Arts Entertainment-Education for HIV/AIDS Prevention and Health Promotion: Practice and Research." *Journal of Health Communication* no 7.1 (2002): 39-57.

Participatory Theatre: A Blended Methodology

2. Rifkin, F. *The Ethics of Participatory Theatre in Higher Education: A Framework for Learning and Teaching.* The Higher Education Academy, Palatine Dance, Drama and Music, 2010. http://rltperformingarts.org/newwordpresssite/wp-content/uploads/2018/10/Ethics_of_participatory_theatre.pdf

3. Davis, J.H., Behm, T. "Terminology of drama/theatre with and for children." *Children's Theatre Review* no 27.1 (1978), p. 10-11.

4. Ward, W. *Playmaking with children from kindergarten through junior high school* (2d ed.). New York: Appleton-Century-Crofts, 1957.

5. Heathcote, D. "Drama as a Process for Change." In *Twentieth-century Theatre: A Sourcebook*, edited by Richard Drain 199-201. London ; New York: Routledge, 1995.

6. Boal, Augusto. *Theatre of the Oppressed*. New York: Urizen, 1979.

7. Huxley, M., & Witts, N. *The Twentieth-century performance reader*. New York: Routledge, 1996.

8. Freire, Paulo. *Pedagogy of the Oppressed*. London: Penguin, 1972.

9. Huxley, M., & Witts, N. *The Twentieth-century Performance Reader*. New York: Routledge, 1996.

10. Kandil, Y. "Participatory Theatre." *The SAGE Encyclopedia of Action Research* (2014): I-Y. 609-610.

11. For more on this line of thought, see:

Alston, A. *Beyond Immersive Theatre: Aesthetics, Politics and Productive Participation*. London: Palgrave, 2016.

Macmillan and Worthen, W. "The written troubles of the brain": Sleep No More and the Space of Character. *Theatre Journal* 64, no. 1 (2012): 79-97.

Game + Story = Participatory Theatre

12. Flanagan, Mary. *Critical Play: Radical Game Design*. Cambridge, MA: MIT, 2009.

13. Squire, Kurt, and Henry Jenkins. "Harnessing the Power of Games in Education." *Insight* 3, no. 1 (2003): 7-31. https://www.semanticscholar.org/paper/HARNESSING-THE-POWER-OF-GAMES-IN-EDUCATION-Squire-Jenkins/718e12db4a77643b1584419eaa8983c655cbf5f9

The 4 Ps of Participatory Theatre

14. Glik, Deborah, Glen Nowak, Thomas Valente, Karena Sapsis, and Chad Martin. "Youth Performing Arts Entertainment-Education for HIV/AIDS Prevention and Health Promotion: Practice and Research." *Journal of Health Communication* 7, no. 1 (2002): 39-57.

15. Spolin, Viola. *Theater Games for the Classroom: A Teacher's Handbook*. Evanston, IL: Northwestern UP, 1986.

16. Rossiter, Kate, Pia Kontos, Angela Colantonio, Julie Gilbert, Julia Gray, and Michelle Keightley. "Staging Data: Theatre as a Tool for Analysis and Knowledge Transfer in Health Research." *Social Science & Medicine* 66, no. 1 (2008): 130-46.

17. Bates, R. A. "Popular theatre: A Useful Process for Adult Educators." *Adult Education Quarterly* 46, no. 4 (1996): 224-36.

How to Use These Activities

18. To access the National Sex Education Standards, visit: https://advocatesforyouth.org/media/future-of-sex-education-national-sex-education-standards-second-edition/

19. We learned this three-part process from Elizabeth Johnson and our colleagues at Liz Lerman's Dance Exchange.

20. Madson, Patricia Ryan. *Improv Wisdom: Don't Prepare, Just Show up*. New York: Bell Tower, 2005.

Chapter 2

21. This activity is adapted from a practice we learned from Elizabeth Johnson and our colleagues at Liz Lerman's Dance Exchange.

www.ingramcontent.com/pod-product-compliance
Lightning Source LLC
Chambersburg PA
CBHW080404270326
41927CB00015B/3340